Peter's Healing Salves

By

Peter

Copyright © 2023 by – Peter – All Rights Reserved.

It is not legal to reproduce, duplicate, or transmit any part of this document in either electronic means or printed format. Recording of this publication is strictly prohibited.

Table of Contents

Disclaimer: i
About the Author ii
Introduction 1
Proper Wound Care 3
Burn Wounds 6
    Peter's Ordinary-Wound Healing Salve: 9
    Peter's Burn-Wound Healing Salve: 13
    Peter's Infected-Wound Healing Salve: 18
    Peter's Burned Infection-Wound Healing Salve: 23
    Potential Compositions for Peter's Burned Infection-Wound Healing Salve: 27
Summary of the Wound Healing Process 31
    Stages of Wound Healing: 34
Purposes of the Healing Salve Ingredients........................ 37
Expectations of the Wound Healing Salves 43
    Peter's Ordinary-Wound Healing Salve   43
    Peter's Burn-Wound Healing Salve   44
    Peter's Infected-Wound Healing Salve   45
    Peter's Burned Infection-Wound Healing Salve   45
Supporting Sources 46

Disclaimer:

For any and all legal purposes, this document is to present my informational opinion only and is NOT intended to treat, cure, or diagnose any illness, wound, disease, etc. I am NOT a medical doctor and have no formal education beyond a high school diploma. According to the online research that I have done, I believe that this information is accurate and will be of great use to people, so long as: it is appropriately modified according to the wound, the wound itself is cleaned appropriately before salve application, the wound receives any other necessary treatment (such as stitches) appropriate to the wound, the salve is prepared in a sanitary manner, and the wound continues to be treated appropriately. All infected wounds, wounds that may have Clostridium tetani (tetanus-causing bacteria), wounds that require stitches, deep wounds, and wounds that bleed a lot (including head wounds) should go to a licensed medical doctor! I extremely highly encourage that such wounds be seen by a licensed medical doctor, quickly. If a doctor recommends that you do NOT use the wound salve, please listen to your doctor and do not use this wound salve. My personal opinion is that this wound salve and the other information in this document could be of great use to people if followed appropriately. If you desire a medical expert's opinion on the information in this book, feel free to consult a licensed medical doctor; I specifically recommend either a licensed naturopathic doctor and/or a dermatologist because they were required to complete coursework specifically relating to this subject that other doctors were not required to complete.

About the Author

I am 25 years old, but I discovered that I love to learn from a very early age. I imagine my elementary school teachers were amused with all I shared with them, which often included the information I obtained from the books in the library. I only discovered how much fun fiction books could be after I had finished reading every nonfiction book in the school library partway through the 3rd grade. However, as I grew older, various people I know have had several major health problems; this directed my learning path into a much more medically-centered one. This book, in particular, was started because my dad was about to have part of his neck fused due to disk issues; that surgery requires a surgical procedure that would cut open at least a foot along his neck and upper back. In preparation for the surgery, I designed my Ordinary-Wound Healing Salve. After sharing some of my salve that I had made with my friends, they suggested I make a book about it. Knowing that it would be beneficial generally, but not for cases of burns and infections, I did further research and designed the other salves at the start of creating this book. There are other medical issues I intend to write about, but this is the subject I am starting with.

Research comes to me very naturally from experience and taking classes in high school and middle school that help me along this path. I was about 14 years old when I first started delving into research papers, such as those found in ncbi, scientific journal, frontiersin.org, etc. At first it took me a few days to understand the full contents of a single research paper as I often had to google things, especially jargon and referenced anatomical pieces - such as nerve cell sections to include the axon and dendrite, specifics of apoptosis, and so on. Thankfully, as time has passed and as I continue to read many more research papers, I can understand them much more easily and faster, especially in a subject I am already familiar with. As far as the schooling goes, a small portion of the things I learned that helped me in this endeavor pertain to assisting me in using a search engine like that of google. For example: +item -thing in google would mean to look for things that contain the keyword item and to exclude the keyword thing, quotations mean looking for that exact phrase, and a colon means to look for that domain address (:ncbi means to look for something from ncbi).

Having lived for 25 years, loving to learn for at least most of that time, and being an avid reader has given me a decent variety of knowledge. This variety enables me to amuse my coworkers from time to time by giving fun facts if they want to hear one, typically about a subject of their choosing.

Introduction

This tiny book primarily focuses on topically applied mixtures that enhance the healing of an injury to the skin, muscles, and blood vessels. These mixtures comprise several ingredients that have been studied individually and occasionally in pairs. Still, I do not know of any current studies combining all of the ingredients listed. Hence, although the individual effects of the ingredients are proven, all of the synergistically enhanced effects are according to my logically-derived beliefs. This book also contains basic wound-care information.

Do NOT ingest these wound-healing salves! They are intended for external use only. Ingestion of relatively high amounts is poisonous! As far as its usage, it should enhance the healing rate and healing quality of the skin, blood vessels, and muscles. It may possibly assist the healing process of nerves and ligaments. It almost certainly will not assist in the healing process of bones. Much of what I state it could heal is deduced by me according to the research papers I have read on the methods in which these things heal the body, individually, and so it is according to my conjecture that the combinations of the ingredients will result in such a positive manner.

In the process of creating the salves, a lot of mixing is required; if one so desires, one can use a couple of small blenders to reduce the mixing time and effort, but blender time varies. The principle is to mix things thoroughly. Liquid sunflower lecithin has a difficult time mixing with water-based things as it prefers bonding to oils, so it takes extra time to mix well with water-based things. Petroleum Jelly is very viscous, making it very hard to mix with oils despite being oil-based, so it requires additional mixing time. When mixing the water-based (with liquid sunflower lecithin) with the oil-based components, it needs more mixing time to ensure the water-bonded sunflower lecithin is able to properly bond with the oils, which will suspend the water-based components in the oil-based components.

Most wound healing salves will last up to 9 months if managed properly, but if the mixture has fresh garlic juice, it will only last up to 72 hours (3 days) because the benefits of fresh garlic juice gradually degrade over 96 hours of it being made (4 days).

For the ingredients, use extra virgin olive oil, cold-pressed coconut oil, extra virgin avocado oil, and cold-pressed aloe vera for the best healing benefits.

Proper Wound Care

Cleaning the wound BEFORE applying any wound-healing salve is essential. Material that is not native to the injured location, except for anything both intentionally and surgically added (like a metal bar and screws, a scaffold to improve healing, stitches, etc), should not remain in the wound. Healing over non-native things, such as a sliver of wood, will almost certainly cause pain, swelling, and infection, even if delayed until after being healed over. Normal cleaning should be gently done with soap and water, and then be gently dried. If applied after a surgery, the surgeons should have cleaned and dried the area before and after the surgery.

Suppose the wound is caused by something with high risk for tetanus-causing bacteria. In that case, you MUST remove all material that shouldn't be there and then thoroughly clean the wound and surrounding tissue with a very generous amount of Hydrogen Peroxide, as quickly after the injury as possible. I specify hydrogen peroxide and not rubbing alcohol because although both are safe to use on open wounds, rubbing alcohol is unable to kill that specific bacteria. In contrast, hydrogen peroxide is able to kill that specific bacteria. The sooner the wound with a high risk of tetanus-causing bacteria is cleaned with hydrogen peroxide, the less time the bacteria will have to reproduce and move deeper into the body. Tetanus-causing bacteria, Clostridium tetani, is found deep within the soil and also within animal intestines. There is a high risk of Clostridium tetani infection if an open wound touches any of the following: unclean animal intestines, animal poop, metal rusted because of being left outside and exposed to the elements *(extremely likely to have been pooped on)*, and metal deep within the soil. If wounded with a high risk of Clostridium tetani (such as on rusted metal listed previously), and you do not have hydrogen peroxide available, allow the wound to bleed a little prior to cleaning and applying something to stop the bleeding. By allowing the wound to bleed, fresh blood can clear out the contaminated blood. Although, if the wound is very serious, causing a great risk of bleeding out (such as an arterial puncture or tear), you should stop the bleeding immediately. In such cases, the person will almost certainly have bled out enough to remove the contaminated blood anyways before you can get to them and stop the bleeding. An iodine solution with a sufficient concentration (at least 5% iodine) is also able to kill Clostridium tetani but is less common and carries more innate risk than hydrogen peroxide.

After applying a wound-healing salve on small wounds that are not still bleeding, covering the wound, such as with a band-aid, is likely unnecessary. After applying a healing salve on a burn (there is a specified burn healing salve), including sunburn, the burn is not recommended to be covered unless either a doctor or immediate circumstances require it to be covered. After applying this salve on a still bleeding wound, covering the wound, such as with a band-aid (or gauze pad if necessary), is required. After surgery, ask the doctor when it would be ok to apply the appropriate wound-healing salve on the surgical site.

<u>When taking care of any wound, it is important to keep the wound clean</u>. After the wound is initially cleaned, it should be dressed with an antibacterial ointment, such as one of my wound-healing salves.

Keeping the wound moist reduces ending-scar size, and increases the ability for the body's healing components to move to their designated locations. However, moisture also provides a better environment for bacteria that would cause infection, raising the risk of infection. Antibacterial components should be included to gain the benefits of wound moisture while deterring infection. My wound-healing salves provide both moisturizing and antibacterial components.

Burn Wounds

Burn wounds are divided into 4 types and 3 categories. The 4 types are Radiation (sunburn is an example), Thermal (heat-caused, such as from fire, stovetop, hot water, etc), Electrical, and Chemical (such as from corrosive chemicals). The 3 categories are listed as 1, 2, or 3 severity. Severity 1 is a simple burn resulting in cell death only in the top layer of skin (epidermis). Severity 2 is a moderately deep burn resulting in cell death in 2 layers of skin (epidermis and dermis); this type will develop blisters. Severity 3 is a deep burn resulting in cell death in all 3 layers of skin (epidermis, dermis, and hypodermis); this usually presents itself as blackened skin and numbness or lack of pain in the worst areas of the burn. <u>The amount of skin burned and the severity of those burns greatly affect the risk factors of fluid loss and body temperature control</u>. The worse the severity, the worse the fluid loss rate, and the more skin affected, the more area for the loss. Any severity 1 burns that are over 70% of the skin area should see the patient in the Emergency Room. Any severity 2 burns over 30% of the skin area should see the patient in the Emergency Room. Any severity 3 burns whatsoever should see the patient in the Emergency Room. Also, if there is swelling in the burned areas, go to the Emergency Room. If it is a chemical burn of any size and severity, go to the Emergency Room. Not meeting these danger criteria does not diminish other things that would cause someone to need to go to the emergency room - for example, a 1st degree burn over 5% of the skin area and a rattlesnake bite, the patient should immediately go to the Emergency Room, not because of the burn, but because of the rattlesnake bite.

For reference, the general consensus of skin area percentages for a non-obese adult is: chest 9%, stomach 9%, upper back 9%, lower back 9%, front half of the arm 4.5% each, back half of the arm 4.5% each, front half of each leg 9%, back half of each leg 9%, total head and neck 9%, genitals 1%. For non-obese children, the general consensus is chest 9%, stomach 9%, upper back 9%, lower back 9%, front half of the arm 4.5% each, back half of the arm 4.5% each, front half of each leg 8%, back half of each leg 8%, total head and neck 13%, genitals 1%. The younger the child, the more the head percentage, reducing the percentage of the legs, with the most extreme being infants, with 17% of the skin being the head, with 7% for the front and 7% for the back of each leg. The leg includes the foot, and the arm includes the hand. Obesity sees the stomach and chest take a slightly larger percentage, reducing the percentage for the arms, legs, head, and neck. These are rough estimates ONLY.

Chemical burns have a high risk of further damage by the direct action of the chemical, which is not limited to potential poisoning, and is in addition to the damage done to the skin. The burn severity and extensivities listed as the cause for going to the hospital is because those are the generalized amounts for established dangerous levels of risks, which include: hypovolemic shock *(the rapid and extensive loss of fluid resulting in shock)*, traumatic shock *(the severity and extensiveness of the injury resulting in shock)*, hypothermia *(too low body heat)*, potential of loss of limb *(treatment may include skin grafting)*, severe inflammatory reaction *(not very different, in effect, to anaphylactic shock)*, pain *(which also causes numerous involuntary bodily reactions that impede the healing process)*, and infection. The risk of hypothermia is because internal body heat leaves the body much faster through burn wounds than through normal skin or even small ordinary injuries.

The first step of burn wound care is to remove the person from the cause, whether that is putting them in the shade, away from the electrical source, cleaning off the chemical *(with clean water and soap)*, etc. The second step of burn wound care is maintaining the hydration of the patient, as the burn injury can cause a lot of fluid loss; this step should be continued during steps 2-5. To hydrate the patient, use electrolyte-enhanced water, such as gatorade or powerade, at least all the way through step 4 and perhaps a little into step 5. Electrolytes manage many things concerning cells, including water management in and out of cells and blood vessels, as well as action potential and activation. The third step is to evaluate the severity of the situation: should the person go to the hospital? The fourth step is to cool down the burn, which is typically done by running cool (but not cold) water over the burn for several minutes (some research indicated a full 20 minutes). The 5th step is prolonged wound care, such as periodic cleaning and application of a healing salve (please note that THIS is the point of salve application, which is after the burn is cooled). If the result of step three is taking the patient to the hospital, then go to the hospital where they will take care of step 4 and a portion of step 5. Going to the hospital does not guarantee survival, but it does greatly improve the chance of survival. Be on the lookout for heat exhaustion and heat stroke, as they can also cause major complications (and heat stroke can cause death), especially in relation to sunburn.

This is my informational opinion ONLY and should not be construed as medical advice from a medical professional.

Peter's Ordinary-Wound Healing Salve:

Composition: Coconut Oil 18%, Olive Oil 18%, Avocado Oil 16%, Aloe Vera 15%, White Petroleum Jelly 9%, Liquid Sunflower Lecithin 8%, Calendula Alcoholic Extract 7% (~70% Calendula), Eucalyptus EO 3%, Tea Tree EO 3%, Peppermint EO 3%. <u>This salve should be applied every 12 hours, with a gentle cleaning and drying once daily.</u> **DO NOT EAT OR DRINK THIS HEALING SALVE!**

Small quantity ~4oz, <u>1% = 0.25 tsp</u>: Aloe Vera 3.75 tsp, Calendula Alcoholic Extract 1.75 tsp, Liquid Sunflower Lecithin 2 tsp, Coconut Oil 4.5 tsp, Olive Oil 4.5 tsp, Avocado Oil 4 tsp, White Petroleum Jelly 2.25 tsp, Eucalyptus EO 0.75 tsp, Tea Tree EO 0.75 tsp, Peppermint EO 0.75 tsp.

Medium quantity ~8oz, <u>1% = 0.5 tsp</u>: Aloe Vera 7.5 tsp, Calendula Alcoholic Extract 3.5 tsp, Liquid Sunflower Lecithin 4 tsp, Coconut Oil 9 tsp, Olive Oil 9 tsp, Avocado Oil 8 tsp, White Petroleum Jelly 4.5 tsp, Eucalyptus EO 1.5 tsp, Tea Tree EO 1.5 tsp, Peppermint EO 1.5 tsp.

Large quantity ~16oz, <u>1% = 1 tsp</u>: Aloe Vera 15 tsp, Calendula Alcoholic Extract 7 tsp, Liquid Sunflower Lecithin 8 tsp, Coconut Oil 18 tsp, Olive Oil 18 tsp, Avocado Oil 16 tsp, White Petroleum Jelly 9 tsp, Eucalyptus EO 3 tsp, Tea Tree EO 3 tsp, Peppermint EO 3 tsp.

Step 1: Mix the Aloe Vera and Calendula Alcoholic Extract together into bowl 1 with wire whisk 1 for about 5 seconds. *(Would also include water-based antiseptics, NOT like polysporin or neosporin.)*

Step 2: Add the Liquid Sunflower Lecithin into bowl 1. Mix thoroughly with wire whisk 1, which means at least 1 minute, to ensure the Sunflower Lecithin is bonded to the water-based components.

Step 3: Add everything else (*all the oils*) except for the White Petroleum Jelly into bowl 2 and mix well with wire whisk 2 for at least 30 seconds. *(Coconut oil, Olive oil, Avocado oil, Eucalyptus EO, Tea Tree EO, and Peppermint EO; would also include Lavender EO, Clove EO, and oil/petroleum-based antiseptics like polysporin.)* If anything needs melted (such as the coconut oil), use a slow introduction of heat, and do NOT use a microwave.

Step 4: Add White Petroleum Jelly into bowl 2 and mix super thoroughly with wire whisk 2, which means at least 180 seconds.

Step 5: Add the contents of bowl 1 into bowl 2; then stir them together thoroughly, with either whisk, for at least 2 minutes.

Step 6: Store in a closed container (closed container: a lidded container with the lid closed). Do not freeze; do not raise the salve's temperature above 110°F; store away from light, such as a cupboard or in a fridge; especially do not expose to ultraviolet light, such as from sunlight, tanning lights, fluorescent lights, UV lights, and plant-

growing lights. Do not microwave. This salve will last up to 9 months after preparation.

Immediately Before Use: Stir contents with a wire whisk for at least 30 seconds to remix any separated components.

During and After Use: Do not contaminate the mixture, such as with bodily fluids (including blood), mold spores (such as by opening it with mold nearby), etc. When using the salve, please pour the desired amount into a separate container or scoop it out with a spoon or something similar.

Specific Use: <u>This is the salve for most wounds</u>. If a burn wound, see Peter's Burn-Wound Healing Salve. If an already infected wound, or a wound very likely to become infected - like a shark bite - use Peter's Infected-Wound Healing Salve. Burn wounds caused by electricity or chemicals should use this salve. If chemically caused, be certain to remove ALL of the harmful chemicals and get approval from a doctor prior to ANY use of this salve! Use Peter's Burned Infection-Wound Healing Salve if an already-infected wound was recently burned.

Allergies to Essential Oils:

If you are allergic to any ONE of the following: Peppermint Essential Oil, Eucalyptus Essential Oil, or Tea Tree Essential Oil, please replace the EO you are allergic to with the other two EO's evenly. For example: instead of Eucalyptus EO 0.75 tsp (3%), Tea Tree EO 0.75

tsp (3%), Peppermint EO 0.75 tsp (3%), you could do Eucalyptus EO 1.125 tsp (4.5%), Tea Tree EO 1.125 tsp (4.5%).

If you are allergic to 2 of the essential oils, please increase the EO you are not allergic to by 50%, and replace the remaining amount of the EOs with an antiseptic, such as polysporin or neosporin. For example: instead of Eucalyptus EO 0.75 tsp (3%), Tea Tree EO 0.75 tsp (3%), Peppermint EO 0.75 tsp (3%), you could do Peppermint EO 1.125 tsp (4.5%) and Polysporin 1.125 tsp (4.5%).

If you are allergic to all 3 of the essential oils, please replace them with 1 or more antiseptics, such as polysporin, neosporin, bacitracin, etc, to account for all 9% that the essential oils have in the composition. Please realize that by replacing the essential oils with antiseptics, you do keep the antibacterial aspect of the mixture, but you still lose the other benefits of the essential oils.

This is my informational opinion ONLY and should not be construed as medical advice from a medical professional.

Peter's Burn-Wound Healing Salve:

Composition: Coconut Oil 10%, Olive Oil 15%, Avocado Oil 15%, Aloe Vera 25%, White Petroleum Jelly 5%, Liquid Sunflower Lecithin 12%, Calendula Alcoholic Extract 7% (~70% Calendula), Eucalyptus EO 5%, Tea Tree EO 2%, Peppermint EO 4%. <u>This salve should be applied about every 6-9 hours, with gentle cleaning and drying once per day.</u> **DO NOT EAT OR DRINK THIS HEALING SALVE!**

Small quantity ~4oz, <u>1% = 0.25 tsp</u>: Aloe Vera 6.25 tsp, Calendula Alcoholic Extract 1.75 tsp, Liquid Sunflower Lecithin 3 tsp, Coconut Oil 2.5 tsp, Olive Oil 3.75 tsp, Avocado Oil 3.75 tsp, White Petroleum Jelly 1.25 tsp, Eucalyptus EO 1.25 tsp, Tea Tree EO 0.5 tsp, Peppermint EO 1 tsp.

Medium quantity ~8oz, <u>1% = 0.5 tsp</u>: Aloe Vera 12.5 tsp, Calendula Alcoholic Extract 3.5 tsp, Liquid Sunflower Lecithin 6 tsp, Coconut Oil 5 tsp, Olive Oil 7.5 tsp, Avocado Oil 7.5 tsp, White Petroleum Jelly 2.5 tsp, Eucalyptus EO 2.5 tsp, Tea Tree EO 1 tsp, Peppermint EO 2 tsp.

Large quantity ~16oz, <u>1% = 1 tsp</u>: Aloe Vera 25 tsp, Calendula Alcoholic Extract 7 tsp, Liquid Sunflower Lecithin 12 tsp, Coconut Oil 10 tsp, Olive Oil 15 tsp, Avocado Oil 15 tsp, White Petroleum Jelly 5 tsp, Eucalyptus EO 5 tsp, Tea Tree EO 2 tsp, Peppermint EO 4 tsp.

Step 1: Mix the Aloe Vera and Calendula Alcoholic Extract together into bowl 1 with wire whisk 1 for about 5 seconds. *(Would also include water-based antiseptics, NOT like polysporin or neosporin.)*

Step 2: Add the Liquid Sunflower Lecithin into bowl 1. Mix thoroughly with wire whisk 1, which means at least 1 minute, to ensure the Sunflower Lecithin is bonded to the water-based components.

Step 3: Add everything else (*all the oils*) except for the White Petroleum Jelly into bowl 2 and mix well with wire whisk 2 for at least 30 seconds. *(Coconut oil, Olive oil, Avocado oil, Eucalyptus EO, Tea Tree EO, and Peppermint EO; would also include Lavender EO, and oil/petroleum-based antiseptics like polysporin.)* If anything needs melting (such as the coconut oil), use a slow introduction of heat, and do NOT use a microwave.

Step 4: Add White Petroleum Jelly into bowl 2 and mix super thoroughly with wire whisk 2, which means at least 180 seconds.

Step 5: Add the contents of bowl 1 into bowl 2; then stir them together thoroughly, with either whisk, for at least 2 minutes.

Step 6: Store in a closed container (closed container: a lidded container with the lid closed). Do not freeze; do not raise the salve's temperature above 110°F; store away from light, such as a cupboard or in a fridge; especially do not expose to ultraviolet light, such as from sunlight, tanning lights, fluorescent lights, UV lights, and plant-

growing lights. Do not microwave. This salve will last up to 9 months after preparation.

Immediately Before Use: Stir contents with a wire whisk for at least 30 seconds to remix any separated components.

During and After Use: Do not contaminate the mixture, such as with bodily fluids (including blood), mold spores (such as by opening it with mold nearby), etc. When using the salve, please pour the desired amount into a separate container or scoop it out with a spoon or something similar. Prior to using this salve for the 1st time on a recent burn, ensure the wound is already cooled!

Specific Use: This mixture is intended to help the initial process of healing of burn wounds from only <u>radiation (including sunburn) and thermal (heat) burns</u>; <u>*NOT chemical or electrical burns*</u>. This salve is designed to assist the body in regaining thermoregulation in the injured area by not trapping in heat, promoting blood flow to the region, and stimulating a cooling sensation. <u>After 24 hours from being burned, use Peter's Ordinary-Wound Healing Salve unless the burn is still overheated.</u> This mixture is NOT to be used for chemical or electrical burns. For electrical burns, use Peter's Ordinary-Wound Healing Salve instead. For chemical burns, ONLY AFTER the wound is completely cleared of the harmful chemical, and also after a doctor says it is ok for you to use a healing salve on the wound, THEN use Peter's Ordinary-Wound Healing Salve. Friction burns are not considered as actual burns in relation to these salves, so for friction burns use Peter's Ordinary-Wound Healing Salve.

Allergies to Essential Oils:

If you are allergic to Peppermint EO, but not allergic to Eucalyptus EO or Tea Tree EO, then change them from Eucalyptus EO 5%, Peppermint EO 4%, Tea Tree EO 2% to Eucalyptus EO 8%, no Peppermint EO, Tea Tree EO 3%.

If you are allergic to Tea Tree EO, but not allergic to Eucalyptus EO or Peppermint EO, then change them from Eucalyptus EO 5%, Peppermint EO 4%, Tea Tree EO 2% to Eucalyptus EO 6%, Peppermint EO 5%, no Tea Tree EO.

If you are allergic to Eucalyptus EO, but not allergic to Peppermint EO or Tea Tree EO, then change them from Eucalyptus EO 5%, Peppermint EO 4%, Tea Tree EO 2% to no Eucalyptus EO, Peppermint EO 7%, Tea Tree EO 4%.

If you are allergic to Peppermint and Tea Tree EOs, but not to allergic to Eucalyptus EO, then change them from Eucalyptus EO 5%, Peppermint EO 4%, Tea Tree EO 2% to Eucalyptus EO 8%, no Peppermint EO, no Tea Tree EO, Antiseptic (such as polysporin or neosporin, etc) 3%.

If you are allergic to Eucalyptus and Tea Tree EOs, but not allergic to Peppermint EO, then change them from Eucalyptus EO 5%, Peppermint EO 4%, Tea Tree EO 2% to no Eucalyptus EO, Peppermint EO 8%, no Tea Tree EO, Antiseptic (such as polysporin or neosporin, etc) 3%.

If you are allergic to Peppermint and Eucalyptus EOs, but not allergic to Tea Tree EO, then change them from Eucalyptus EO 5%, Peppermint EO 4%, Tea Tree EO 2%, Aloe Vera 25%, Liquid Sunflower Lecithin 12% to no Eucalyptus EO, no Peppermint EO, Tea Tree EO 5%, Antiseptic (such as polysporin or neosporin, etc) 3%, Aloe Vera 27%, Liquid Sunflower Lecithin 13%.

If you are allergic to all 3 EOs, then remove the EOs and replace them with Antiseptic (such as polysporin or neosporin, etc) 8%, change Aloe Vera from 25% to 27%, and change Liquid Sunflower Lecithin from 12% to 13%.

This is my informational opinion ONLY and should not be construed as medical advice from a medical professional.

Peter's Infected-Wound Healing Salve:

Composition: Coconut Oil 18%, Olive Oil 15%, Avocado Oil 15%, Aloe Vera 15%, White Petroleum Jelly 4%, Liquid Sunflower Lecithin 8%, Calendula Alcoholic Extract 7% (~70% Calendula), Eucalyptus EO 5%, Tea Tree EO 5%, Peppermint EO 5%, Clove EO 3%. This salve should be applied about every 6-9 hours, with a gentle cleaning and drying immediately prior to every application. **DO NOT EAT OR DRINK THIS HEALING SALVE!**

Small quantity ~4oz, 1% = 0.25 tsp: Aloe Vera 3.75 tsp, Calendula Alcoholic Extract 1.75 tsp, Liquid Sunflower Lecithin 2 tsp, Coconut Oil 4.5 tsp, Olive Oil 3.75 tsp, Avocado Oil 3.75 tsp, White Petroleum Jelly 1 tsp, Eucalyptus EO 1.25 tsp, Tea Tree EO 1.25 tsp, Peppermint EO 1.25 tsp, Clove EO 0.75 tsp.

Medium quantity ~8oz, 1% = 0.5 tsp: Aloe Vera 7.5 tsp, Calendula Alcoholic Extract 3.5 tsp, Liquid Sunflower Lecithin 4 tsp, Coconut Oil 9 tsp, Olive Oil 7.5 tsp, Avocado Oil 7.5 tsp, White Petroleum Jelly 2 tsp, Eucalyptus EO 3 tsp, Tea Tree EO 3 tsp, Peppermint EO 3 tsp, Clove EO 1.5 tsp.

Large quantity ~16oz, 1% = 1 tsp: Aloe Vera 15 tsp, Calendula Alcoholic Extract 7 tsp, Liquid Sunflower Lecithin 8 tsp, Coconut Oil 18 tsp, Olive Oil 15 tsp, Avocado Oil 15 tsp, White Petroleum Jelly 4 tsp, Eucalyptus EO 6 tsp, Tea Tree EO 6 tsp, Peppermint EO 6 tsp, Clove EO 3 tsp.

Step 1: Mix the Aloe Vera and Calendula Alcoholic Extract together into bowl 1 with wire whisk 1 for about 5 seconds. *(Would also include water-based antiseptics, NOT like polysporin or neosporin.)*

Step 2: Add the Liquid Sunflower Lecithin into bowl 1. Mix thoroughly with wire whisk 1, which means at least 1 minute, to ensure the Sunflower Lecithin is bonded to the water-based components.

Step 3: Add everything else (*all the oils*) except for the White Petroleum Jelly into bowl 2 and mix well with wire whisk 2, which means at least 30 seconds. *(Coconut oil, Olive oil, Avocado oil, Eucalyptus EO, Tea Tree EO, and Peppermint EO; would also include Clove EO, and oil/petroleum-based antiseptics like polysporin.)* If anything needs melting (such as the coconut oil), use a slow introduction of heat, and do NOT use a microwave.

Step 4: Add White Petroleum Jelly into bowl 2 and mix super thoroughly with wire whisk 2, which means at least 180 seconds.

Step 5: Add the contents of bowl 1 into bowl 2; then stir them together thoroughly, with either whisk, for at least 2 minutes.

Step 6: Store in a closed container (closed container: a lidded container with the lid closed). Do not freeze; do not raise the salve's temperature above 110°F; store away from light, such as a cupboard or in a fridge; especially do not expose to ultraviolet light, such as from sunlight, tanning lights, fluorescent lights, UV lights, and plant-

growing lights. Do not microwave. This salve will last up to 9 months after preparation.

Immediately Before Use: Stir contents with a wire whisk for at least 30 seconds to remix any separated components.

During and After Use: Do not contaminate the mixture, such as with bodily fluids (to include blood), mold spores (such as by opening it with mold nearby), etc. When using the salve, please pour the desired amount into a separate container or scoop it out with a spoon or something similar.

Specific Use: This salve is intended to fight infection in an infected wound or in a wound with a high risk of becoming infected. If a radiation burn (including sunburn) or thermal burn (from heat, including fire, hot water, stovetop, etc) occurs on an infected burn, use Peter's Burned Infection-Wound Healing Salve. After the infection has been gone for at least 72 hours, use Peter's Ordinary-Wound Healing Salve instead.

Allergies to Essential Oils:

If you are allergic to any ONE of the following: Peppermint Essential Oil, Eucalyptus Essential Oil, or Tea Tree Essential Oil, please replace it 20% with clove, 40% with one of the other EOs, and 40% with the last EO. For example: instead of Peppermint EO 1.25 tsp (5%), Eucalyptus EO 1.25 tsp (5%), Tea Tree 1.25 tsp (5%), and

Clove 0.75 tsp (3%), you can do Eucalyptus 1.75 tsp (7%), Tea Tree 1.75 tsp (7%), and Clove 1 tsp (4%).

If you are allergic to Clove EO, but not the other 3, then replace Clove EO with an antiseptic.

If you are allergic to any TWO of the following: Peppermint EO, Eucalyptus EO, or Tea Tree EO, please replace that amount 20% with an antiseptic, 40% with Clove EO, and 40% with the remaining EO. For example: instead of Peppermint EO 1.25 tsp (5%), Eucalyptus EO 1.25 tsp (5%), Tea Tree 1.25 tsp (5%), and Clove 0.75 tsp (3%), you can do Tea Tree 2.25 tsp (9%), Clove 1.75 tsp (7%), and an antiseptic tsp (2%).

If you are allergic to Clove EO, and 1 of the other 3 EOs, then replace Clove EO with an antiseptic and replace the EO - that you are allergic to - with the 2 EOs you are not allergic to (40% each) and an antiseptic (20%). For example: instead of Peppermint EO 1.25 tsp (5%), Eucalyptus EO 1.25 tsp (5%), Tea Tree 1.25 tsp (5%), and Clove 0.75 tsp (3%), you can do Peppermint EO 1.75 tsp (7%), Eucalyptus EO 1.75 tsp (7%), and an antiseptic 1 tsp (4%).

If you are allergic to 3 of the 4 EOs, then have 10% of the mix be the remaining EO and 8% be an antiseptic. For example: Clove EO 2.5 tsp (10%) and an antiseptic 2 tsp (8%).

If you are allergic to all 4 EOs (equaling 18% of the mixture), then replace about 55% of it (10% of the mixture) with an antiseptic, and about 45% of it (8% of the mixture) with fresh garlic juice. The garlic juice is mixed with the ingredients in step 1. This mixture lasts up to 72 hours after its creation, so I suggest only using the small option.

Obtaining Garlic Juice:

Option 1: peel several cloves of garlic and blend in a small blender with 1/4 of the garlic amount of clean water. After allowing it to sit for 3 minutes, blend again for a few seconds. Allow it to sit for another 3 minutes before straining out solids as best as possible. The remaining liquid is the garlic juice.

Option 2: very finely mince several cloves of garlic and let soak in some clean water equal to 1/4 of the garlic amount, stirring for a second or two every 30 seconds, for 10 minutes. Then strain out all of the solids. The remaining liquid is the garlic juice.

This is my informational opinion ONLY and should not be construed as medical advice from a medical professional.

Peter's Burned Infection-Wound Healing Salve:

An already infected wound got burned.

Composition: Coconut Oil 10%, Olive Oil 13%, Avocado Oil 17%, Aloe Vera 20%, White Petroleum Jelly 2%, Liquid Sunflower Lecithin 9%, Calendula Alcoholic Extract 7% (~70% Calendula), Eucalyptus EO 8%, Tea Tree EO 4%, Peppermint EO 4%, Clove EO 6%. This salve should be applied about every 6 hours, with a mild cleaning and drying immediately prior to every application.

Small quantity ~4oz, 1% = 0.25 tsp: Aloe Vera 5 tsp, Calendula Alcoholic Extract 1.75 tsp, Liquid Sunflower Lecithin 2.25 tsp, Coconut Oil 2.5 tsp, Olive Oil 3.25 tsp, Avocado Oil 4.25 tsp, White Petroleum Jelly 0.5 tsp, Eucalyptus EO 2 tsp, Tea Tree EO 1 tsp, Peppermint EO 1 tsp, Clove EO 1.5 tsp.

Medium quantity ~8oz, 1% = 0.5 tsp: Aloe Vera 10 tsp, Calendula Alcoholic Extract 3.5 tsp, Liquid Sunflower Lecithin 4.5 tsp, Coconut Oil 5 tsp, Olive Oil 6.5 tsp, Avocado Oil 8.5 tsp, White Petroleum Jelly 1 tsp, Eucalyptus EO 4 tsp, Tea Tree EO 2 tsp, Peppermint EO 2 tsp, Clove EO 3 tsp.

Large quantity ~16oz, 1% = 1 tsp: Aloe Vera 20 tsp, Calendula Alcoholic Extract 7 tsp, Liquid Sunflower Lecithin 9 tsp, Coconut Oil 10 tsp, Olive Oil 13 tsp, Avocado Oil 17 tsp, White Petroleum Jelly 2 tsp, Eucalyptus EO 8 tsp, Tea Tree EO 4 tsp, Peppermint EO 4 tsp, Clove EO 6 tsp.

Obtaining Garlic Juice:

Option 1: peel several cloves of garlic and blend in a small blender with 1/4 of the garlic amount of clean water. After allowing it to sit for 3 minutes, blend again for a few seconds. Allow it to sit for another 3 minutes before straining out solids as best as possible. The remaining liquid is the garlic juice.

Option 2: very finely mince several cloves of garlic and let soak in some clean water equal to 1/4 of the garlic amount, stirring for a second or two every 30 seconds, for 10 minutes. Then strain out all of the solids. The remaining liquid is the garlic juice.

Making the Healing Salve:

Step 1: Mix the Aloe Vera, Calendula Alcoholic Extract, and Garlic Juice (if included) together into bowl 1 with wire whisk 1 for about 5 seconds. *(Would also include water-based antiseptics, NOT like polysporin or neosporin.)*

Step 2: Add the Liquid Sunflower Lecithin into bowl 1. Mix thoroughly with wire whisk 1, which means at least 1 minute, to ensure the Sunflower Lecithin is bonded to the water-based components.

Step 3: Add everything else (*all the oils*) except for the White Petroleum Jelly into bowl 2 and mix well with wire whisk 2, which means at least 30 seconds. *(Coconut oil, Olive oil, Avocado oil, Eucalyptus EO, Tea Tree EO, and Peppermint EO; would also include Lavender EO, Clove EO, and oil/petroleum-based antiseptics like polysporin.)* If anything needs melted (such as the coconut oil), use a slow introduction of heat, and do NOT use a microwave.

Step 4: Add White Petroleum Jelly into bowl 2 and mix super thoroughly with wire whisk 2, which means at least 180 seconds.

Step 5: Add the contents of bowl 1 into bowl 2; then stir them together thoroughly, with either whisk, for at least 2 minutes.

Step 6: Store in a closed container (closed container: a lidded container with the lid closed). Do not freeze; do not raise the salve's temperature above 110°F; store away from light, such as a cupboard or in a fridge; especially do not expose to ultraviolet light, such as from sunlight, tanning lights, fluorescent lights, UV lights, and plant-growing lights. Do not microwave. This salve will last up to 9 months after preparation.

Immediately Before Use: Stir contents with a wire whisk for at least 30 seconds to remix any separated components.

During and After Use: Do not contaminate the mixture, such as with bodily fluids (to include blood), mold spores (such as by opening it with mold nearby), etc. When using the salve, please pour the desired amount into a separate container or scoop it out with a spoon or something similar. Prior to using this salve for the 1st time on a recent burn, ensure the burn is already cooled!

Specific Use: This salve is intended to <u>simultaneously treat a recent burn from either radiation (including sunburn) or thermal (heat) and combat infection in an infected wound</u>; *<u>infected wounds that have been electrically burned should use Peter's Infected-Wound Healing Salve</u>* instead of this one; infected wounds that have been chemically burned, ONLY AFTER being thoroughly cleaned and after a doctor clears you to use a healing salve, should use Peter's Infected-Wound Healing Salve instead of this one. This salve mixes aspects of the Burn-Wound Healing Salve and the Infected-Wound Healing Salve, which means high antimicrobial action plus assisting the body in regaining thermoregulation in the injured area. <u>After 24 hours of being burned and after the infection has been removed for at least 72 hours, if the wound is still overheated,</u> use Peter's Ordinary-Wound Healing Salve. After 24 hours of being burned and if the infection has not been gotten rid of for at least 72 hours, unless the burn is still overheated, use Peter's Infected-Wound Healing Salve until the infection has been gone for 72 hours or longer, and then change to Peter's Ordinary-Wound Healing Salve. If the wound has been burned within the past 24 hours and has not been infected for the past 72 hours, then see Peter's Burn-Wound Healing Salve instead of this one. Friction burns are not considered as an actual burn in relation to these salves, so if an infected wound receives a friction burn, use Peter's Infected-Wound Healing Salve instead of this one.

Potential Compositions for Peter's Burned Infection-Wound Healing Salve:

Clove, Peppermint, Eucalyptus, Tea Tree:

Composition: Coconut Oil 10%, Olive Oil 13%, Avocado Oil 17%, Aloe Vera 20%, White Petroleum Jelly 2%, Liquid Sunflower Lecithin 9%, Calendula Alcoholic Extract 7% (~70% Calendula), Eucalyptus EO 8%, Tea Tree EO 4%, Peppermint EO 4%, Clove EO 6%.

Clove, Peppermint, Eucalyptus:

Composition: Coconut Oil 10%, Olive Oil 13%, Avocado Oil 17%, Aloe Vera 20%, White Petroleum Jelly 2%, Liquid Sunflower Lecithin 9%, Calendula Alcoholic Extract 7% (~70% Calendula), Eucalyptus EO 9%, Peppermint EO 5%, Clove EO 8%.

Clove, Peppermint, Tea Tree:

Composition: Coconut Oil 10%, Olive Oil 13%, Avocado Oil 17%, Aloe Vera 24%, White Petroleum Jelly 2%, Liquid Sunflower Lecithin 11%, Calendula Alcoholic Extract 7% (~70% Calendula), Tea Tree EO 4%, Peppermint EO 4%, Clove EO 8%.

Clove, Peppermint:

Composition: Coconut Oil 10%, Olive Oil 13%, Avocado Oil 17%, Aloe Vera 24%, White Petroleum Jelly 2%, Liquid Sunflower Lecithin 11%, Calendula Alcoholic Extract 7% (~70% Calendula),

Peppermint EO 4%, Clove EO 8%, Antiseptic (such as polysporin or neosporin, etc) 4%.

Clove, Eucalyptus, Tea Tree:

Composition: Coconut Oil 10%, Olive Oil 13%, Avocado Oil 17%, Aloe Vera 20%, White Petroleum Jelly 2%, Liquid Sunflower Lecithin 9%, Calendula Alcoholic Extract 7% (~70% Calendula), Eucalyptus EO 9%, Tea Tree EO 5%, Clove EO 8%.

Clove, Eucalyptus:

Composition: Coconut Oil 10%, Olive Oil 13%, Avocado Oil 17%, Aloe Vera 20%, White Petroleum Jelly 2%, Liquid Sunflower Lecithin 9%, Calendula Alcoholic Extract 7% (~70% Calendula), Eucalyptus EO 9%, Clove EO 8%, Antiseptic 5%.

Clove, Tea Tree:

Composition: Coconut Oil 10%, Olive Oil 13%, Avocado Oil 17%, Aloe Vera 24%, White Petroleum Jelly 2%, Liquid Sunflower Lecithin 11%, Calendula Alcoholic Extract 7% (~70% Calendula), Tea Tree EO 3%, Clove EO 8%, Antiseptic 5%.

Peppermint, Eucalyptus, Tea Tree:

Composition: Coconut Oil 10%, Olive Oil 13%, Avocado Oil 17%, Aloe Vera 20%, White Petroleum Jelly 2%, Liquid Sunflower Lecithin 9%, Calendula Alcoholic Extract 7% (~70% Calendula), Eucalyptus EO 8%, Tea Tree EO 4%, Peppermint EO 4%, Antiseptic 6%.

Peppermint, Eucalyptus:

Composition: Coconut Oil 10%, Olive Oil 13%, Avocado Oil 17%, Aloe Vera 20%, White Petroleum Jelly 2%, Liquid Sunflower Lecithin 9%, Calendula Alcoholic Extract 7% (~70% Calendula), Eucalyptus EO 9%, Peppermint EO 5%, Antiseptic 8%.

Peppermint, Tea Tree:

Composition: Coconut Oil 10%, Olive Oil 13%, Avocado Oil 17%, Aloe Vera 24%, White Petroleum Jelly 2%, Liquid Sunflower Lecithin 11%, Calendula Alcoholic Extract 7% (~70% Calendula), Tea Tree EO 4%, Peppermint EO 4%, Antiseptic 8%.

Peppermint:

Composition: Coconut Oil 10%, Olive Oil 13%, Avocado Oil 17%, Aloe Vera 25%, White Petroleum Jelly 2%, Liquid Sunflower Lecithin 11%, Calendula Alcoholic Extract 7% (~70% Calendula), Peppermint EO 6%, Antiseptic 9%.

Eucalyptus, Tea Tree:

Composition: Coconut Oil 10%, Olive Oil 13%, Avocado Oil 17%, Aloe Vera 22%, White Petroleum Jelly 2%, Liquid Sunflower Lecithin 10%, Calendula Alcoholic Extract 7% (~70% Calendula), Eucalyptus EO 8%, Tea Tree EO 4%, Antiseptic 7%.

Eucalyptus:

Composition: Coconut Oil 10%, Olive Oil 13%, Avocado Oil 17%, Aloe Vera 22%, White Petroleum Jelly 2%, Liquid Sunflower Lecithin 10%, Calendula Alcoholic Extract 7% (~70% Calendula), Eucalyptus EO 10%, Antiseptic 9%.

Tea Tree:

Composition: Coconut Oil 10%, Olive Oil 13%, Avocado Oil 17%, Aloe Vera 25%, White Petroleum Jelly 2%, Liquid Sunflower Lecithin 11%, Calendula Alcoholic Extract 7% (~70% Calendula), Tea Tree EO 5%, Antiseptic 10%.

No Essential Oils:

Composition: Coconut Oil 10%, Olive Oil 13%, Avocado Oil 17%, Aloe Vera 25%, White Petroleum Jelly 1%, Liquid Sunflower Lecithin 11%, Calendula Alcoholic Extract 7% (~70% Calendula), Antiseptic 10%, Fresh Garlic Juice 6%. This mixture lasts up to 72 hours after its creation.

This is my informational opinion ONLY and should not be construed as medical advice from a medical professional.

Summary of the Wound Healing Process

There are four overlapping stages to wound healing: Hemostasis, Inflammation, Proliferation, and Restructuring. The Inflammation phase will begin during the Hemostasis phase and end during the Proliferation phase, which in turn will end during the Restructuring phase. The actual duration of each phase varies from wound to wound and is affected by diverse factors.

Term Definitions:

Cytokines: various chemicals and proteins released by cells to communicate to other cells that something is wrong, such as that they are damaged or infected.

Immune Cell: a cell of the immune system and often known as a white blood cell. There are several types of immune cells, and all are involved in policing foreign or damaged compounds, proteins, and cells.

Macrophage: a type of immune cell, and is essentially a cell dump truck. This type of cell is responsible for eating/collecting "trash" and removing it from the body.

Inflammation: Inflammation is a response to cytokines and with a primary result of calling for immune cells. The response to the inflammatory cytokines is to increase fluid in the space between cells, which allows much more movement of things within the tissue.

Proliferation: the reproduction of cells. Cells have a process where they double their inner components and then divide into two identical new cells (well, almost always identical).

Tissue: a group of cells bound together.

Blood Vessel: a tube made up of cells that transports blood inside.

Arteries: blood vessels that take blood away from the heart toward other body areas. Blood has the most pressure once leaving the heart, and so arteries are the blood vessels with the thickest walls.

Veins: blood vessels that take blood toward the heart away from other areas of the body. These are roughly the same size as the arteries, but due to a lower pressure requirement, they have thinner walls than the arteries.

Capillaries: the smallest of blood vessels, and is the actual point where blood exchanges oxygen and other nutrients for cellular waste with the cells between the cells and blood vessels. Capillaries are spread through every tissue of the body.

Fibrin: a protein that does not dissolve in water.

Growth Factors: chemicals and proteins that stimulate the proliferation of cells.

Apoptosis: programmed cell suicide. This occurs to protect the surrounding tissues, and ultimately the organism, when the process within the cell is completed. This process is full of counterbalances and measures to try and identify when the cell is compromised beyond the point of repair. The end result of apoptosis is the complete breakdown of the inside of the cell followed by compaction of the cell to end up as a compact husk with all of the potential causes for harm safely packed inside and away from interacting with the cell's surroundings.

Necrosis: a sudden death and rupture of cells. The cell dies and releases all of its contents into its surroundings.

Epithelium: The outermost layer of a body surface, such as the outer layer of the skin, or of an organ, or of a canal, etc, and it keeps things that are outside on the outside.

Epithelialization: The process of regrowing the Epithelium. In almost all uses of the term, it means healing the outermost layer of the skin.

Angiogenesis: The process of growing new blood vessels, including capillaries.

Inhibit: Slow, restrain, or prevent from happening.

Granulation Tissue: New tissue with many capillaries and quickly proliferating cells throughout it.

Endothelial Cell: The type of cell that creates the inner lining of blood vessels, which is most of the material in capillaries. These cells regulate the exchange of material into and out of blood.

Fibroblasts: The primary cell of the dermis.

Keratinocytes: The primary cell of the epidermis.

Stages of Wound Healing:

Hemostasis: This phase stops blood loss. First, the affected blood vessels constrict, reducing blood flow to the area. Second, platelets form a thin, basic, and soft clot to trap blood and contain it in the area. Third, various chemicals are released by the cells to increase production of binding proteins, including fibrin. Fourth, the blood, platelets, and fibrin are bound together, forming what is known as a blood clot. A dried blood clot is known as a scab.

Inflammation: In this stage, the tissue directly surrounding the wound increases fluid content in the intercellular space (the space in a tissue between the cells) and cells produce cytokines, which call immune cells to the area. During hemostasis, increasing the fluid content (primarily water) reduces the fluid trying to escape the blood vessel, making the blood thicker. After hemostasis, the extra fluid content allows greater movement of immune cells, growth factors, nutrients, and other cells. During this time, immune cells kill and remove foreign and damaged bodies, including bacteria, viruses, fungi, other foreign material, damaged/dead cells, and cellular waste. Too much inflammation results in apoptosis and necrosis of healthy cells and the cytokines signal cells to stop proliferating, which competes with the growth factors trying to cause the cells to proliferate. The primary reason for inflammation is to saturate the tissue with immune cells to clean up the wounded area, which is why an infected wound will also become inflamed.

Proliferation: The primary component of this stage is a large increase in cell proliferation. Also occurring in this phase, various small cell groups are moving into the damaged area, which is inhibited by a dry wound. An essential part of this phase is having the nutrients necessary for the proliferation to occur, which includes proteins, fatty acids, vitamins, minerals, enzymes, and growth factors. This phase closes the wound by the simultaneous use of three methods. In the first method, cells proliferate on the edges of the wound until the edges of the wound grow into each other; this causes a scab to lift. In the second method, small cell groups migrate into parts of the wounded area and rapidly proliferate to fill in the area with new cells. In the third method, cells release binding components that pull the live cells in and around the wound toward each other. Wound closure and epithelialization occur in this stage.

Restructuring: This phase is also known by other names, to include remodeling phase or maturation phase. In the proliferation phase, a variety of cells and connective components that participate in the closing of the wound are mass produced according to the needs of healing and sealing the wound but beyond what is needed in uninjured tissue; in this phase the excess cells undergo apoptosis and are removed alongside the excess connective components. The massive cell proliferation in the proliferation phase requires extra blood vessels to facilitate a much higher transfer load of nutrients and cellular waste; in this phase the extra capillaries undergo a regression phase that closes them off while the now unused capillary cells undergo apoptosis and are removed. As new space is made the cells that remain will shift into a formation that makes a more seamless and functional tissue. Scars are healed wounds that fade away as they are restructured. However, in many instances, tissue will end the restructuring phase before it is 100% restructured, which results in a permanent scar; some causes of this could be the total loss of specific cells that were not replaced early on by the migration of new cells of the same type or interruption or delay of the healing phases.

This is my informational opinion ONLY and should not be construed as medical advice from a medical professional.

Purposes of the Healing Salve Ingredients

Coconut Oil

Coconut oil is moderately antibiotic, has several nutritional components that are often limiting factors in the healing process, and lowers inflammation markers. Although coconut oil has low permeability through the layers of the skin, it does a great job at preventing moisture loss. Coconut oil is best for the epidermis layer.

Coconut oil is great for repairing the skin's water barrier, the epidermis layer, anti-inflammatory action, stimulates cellular proliferation, provides some material for new cell development, and has some antimicrobial effects.

Olive Oil

Olive oil has a lot of nutritional components, more so than coconut oil, that are often limiting factors in the healing process and which are thoroughly used by proliferating cells for material in the proliferation process, in addition to stimulating proliferation. Olive oil, especially because of the high oleic acid content, has high permeability through the layers of the skin, which has positive and negative aspects depending upon the situation. For a positive example, in the case of burn wounds, it increases the flow rate of fluid and nutrients in the tissue; the increased fluid flow rate has a direct thermal equalizing effect. For a negative example, high oleic acid content, due to their tissue penetrating effect, directly interrupts the function of the water barrier of the skin.

Olive oil is a good anti-inflammatory, stimulates cellular proliferation, provides a wealth of material for new cell development, and greatly enhances the flow of fluid and nutrients through the tissue - including the other components in the salve.

Avocado Oil

Avocado oil has more essential fatty acid content than coconut oil but less than olive oil, which means it is between the two in providing material for new cell development. However, it has a large vitamin and mineral impact, many of which affect genetic factors and act as cofactors and catalysts.

Aloe Vera

Aloe vera has several components with diverse cell interactions to stimulate cellular proliferation. Aloe vera, similar to Avocado oil, also has a wealth of vitamins and minerals, though they differ in types and amounts. Aloe vera is also a great source of water. The oils provide a lot of fatty acids that are incorporated into new cells, but Aloe vera provides the water content that is needed; without the water content that Aloe vera provides, that lack would be a limiting factor. This water factor is especially important in burn wounds because heat causes a faster rate of water loss than with normal wounds. Water carries heat away from overheated sections and toward the underheated (cold) sections, creating a heat balancing effect on the tissue, provided there is sufficient fluid movement in the tissue (greatly improved by the Oleic Acid largely in Olive oil and moderately in Avocado oil). If the whole tissue is overheated, it balances the heat but does not actually cool it down beyond evaporative cooling; this is why it is so important to try to cool down the burn prior to application of a burn salve.

White Petroleum Jelly

White petroleum jelly is specifically used to preserve tissue moisture. The retention effect of white petroleum jelly is greater than any of the other components in the salve, but it does not actually add any additional moisture like Aloe vera does, or even to the much lesser extent of Olive, Coconut, and Avocado oils. However, it also has the greatest heat retention effect, with coconut oil being second.

Liquid Sunflower Lecithin

This is an effective emulsifier best used to suspend water into oil, which means the water content should be less than the oil content - which is the case with these salves. Dried sunflower lecithin would be best used to suspend oil into water. This specific emulsifier was used because it has a high capacity effect while also remaining safe for wound treatment. If not for the emulsifier, the oil and water components could not mix to any degree, which would eliminate things like Aloe vera, garlic juice, and any other water-based components.

Calendula Alcoholic Extract

Calendula powerfully stimulates cellular proliferation, including on angiogenesis, exceeding the stimulation of any other component. Coconut oil, Olive oil, Avocado oil, and Aloe vera all work wonders at providing material, cofactors, catalysts, and some cellular proliferation stimulation, but the Calendula easily doubles the stimulation for cellular proliferation. Calendula also modulates genetic expression to influence how they are stimulated to grow, preventing growth in ways that they should not grow (which means this also has antitumor effects).

Eucalyptus Essential Oil

The primary purpose of this oil is as an antimicrobial. However, it also has a beneficial effect on cellular signaling that promotes the healing process. Also, this triggers cold receptors which can reduce uncomfortable feelings such as that of inflammation, and reduces the perception of pain.

Tea Tree Essential Oil

The primary purpose of this oil is as an antimicrobial. However, it also has a mild but still beneficial effect on cellular signaling that promotes the healing process. This oil has different mechanisms of action to the other Essential Oils, which enables the antimicrobial action to act synergistically to the other oils rather than merely cumulatively. This has a stronger antimicrobial action than either Eucalyptus EO or Peppermint EO, but less than Clove EO.

Peppermint Essential Oil

The primary purpose of the oil is to prevent the growth of microbes. There is some bactericidal and fungicidal effect, but the best use of this oil is to prevent the initial presence and proliferation of these various microbes. It also directly stimulates increased cutaneous blood flow (blood flow to the skin). If used with oleic acid, it can help keep an injured area somewhat warmed by sharing the inner body heat due to blood flow, but also by stimulating blood flow it increases exchange rate of nutrients, waste, and cells in the affected area. Furthermore, it has a stimulatory effect upon cells to proliferate, and in a currently unknown mechanism, it also appears to help direct the organization of cells in the tissue, which greatly enhances the remodulation phase.

Clove Essential Oil

Of the essential oils, Clove essential oil has the strongest and best variety of antimicrobial action. However, it also inhibits the production of growth factors from cells. In the case of infection, it does a remarkable job at eliminating the infection, but due to the inhibition of growth factor production, it slightly impairs healing in a non-infection setting.

Fresh Garlic Juice

The primary component of fresh garlic juice is Allicin, one of the greatest antimicrobials, anti-inflammatories, and pro-immune-system I have ever encountered. Whether it does as good or better than Clove EO I am not sure, but I would probably lean toward it being better. The issue with its use is the very short lifespan of Allicin, as it is formed and breaks down into its various post-allicin compounds within a 4 day period, and there is no way to preserve allicin itself from its natural degradation. The post and pre allicin compounds are useful, but at best are only half as useful of an antimicrobial as allicin is. It is not used as the antimicrobial only because of its limited lifespan. In addition to the prodigious antimicrobial effect, it has several other mechanisms that also enhance the healing process.

This is my informational opinion ONLY and should not be construed as medical advice from a medical professional.

Expectations of the Wound Healing Salves

Peter's Ordinary-Wound Healing Salve

I expect this salve to be the primary healing salve, probably being the sole use of 60% or more of wounds. It provides strong antimicrobial action, which means it does well at preventing the most common cause of delayed wound healing. It also provides a wealth of material in the form of water, fatty acids, vitamins, and minerals for cellular reproduction. Additionally, it greatly stimulates cellular proliferation. These things should work together to reduce additional necrosis that typically occurs with recent injuries, improve the influence of the inflammation phase while also reducing the intensity and duration, more than double the activity of the proliferation phase, and assist in the initial action of the restructuring phase. I expect this salve, if used appropriately, to heal wounds at about 300% the speed of healing with just a bandaid or gauze pad covering, in addition to reducing the size and distinctivity of a scar, and preventing at least 70% of infections that would occur. I also have personally experienced a pain-reduction and cooling effect from this salve, which I believe is caused by a mixture of anti-inflammatory action and activation of cold receptors. I do not know if this effect is unique to myself or if it will have the same effect for other people. There are ZERO known tests for this, and also I am NOT a doctor, but this is my informational opinion on the effect of this healing salve.

Peter's Burn-Wound Healing Salve

It is fairly common for burns to not be fully cooled by the conclusion of the cooling period, or to be fully cooled and end up reheating due to coverings, salves, etc, that add or simply retain too much heat in the affected area, or even just that the inflammation phase generates enough heat to cause the burning to resume. This salve is extra rich in water and oleic acid, which should promote the spread of heat in the damaged tissue. By doing this it should reduce bodily response of increasing heat production for cold areas, and also reduce the heat of still heated areas. It should be noted that this effect is more equalizing rather than cooling. Also, by activation of the cooling receptors, it should help in the temperature sensitivity of burn wounds. The reduction of heat-retaining compounds in the ordinary-wound healing salve, namely coconut oil and petroleum jelly, should prevent heat retention. The increase of vitamins and minerals, in addition to extra presence of material for cellular proliferation, should enhance the start of the proliferation phase. The extra activation of the cold receptors and the equalization of the heat in the damaged tissue should result in a soothing sensation to the burned area, and a slightly cold sensation in nearby tissue. The extra water presence early-on in the burn should dramatically reduce the necrosis often experienced in more severe burns. The primary purpose is to instigate an increase of healing while reducing the possibility of residual continuation of tissue damage. I expect this to be the 2nd most-commonly used salve. There are ZERO known tests for this, and also I am NOT a doctor, but this is my informational opinion on the effect of this healing salve.

Peter's Infected-Wound Healing Salve

This particular salve does increase the healing speed, but not as much as the Ordinary-Wound Healing Salve, as the primary focus is eliminating the infection as quickly as possible. The infection itself can be a serious and potentially life-threatening situation, in addition to increasing damage to the wound. The focus of this salve is to eradicate the infection, but the healing rate itself should be a guesstimated 150% of a normal wound, as opposed to the 300% healing rate of the Ordinary-Wound Healing Salve. The signs of infection may be eliminated before the infection is completely eradicated, so continuing with this salve for a small time after the signs are gone is suggested. I expect this to be the 2nd least-commonly used salve. There are ZERO known tests for this, and also I am NOT a doctor, but this is my informational opinion on the effect of this healing salve.

Peter's Burned Infection-Wound Healing Salve

The focus of this salve is to fight the infection. However, the secondary focus is to equalize the heat in the tissue for the purposes mentioned in the section explaining the expectations for the Burn-Wound Healing Salve. In essence, this is a blend of the two salves that are intended for infections or burns specifically. I expect this to be the least-commonly used salve. There are ZERO known tests for this, and also I am NOT a doctor, but this is my informational opinion on the effect of this healing salve.

Supporting Sources

Title: Effect of topical application of virgin coconut oil on skin components and antioxidant status during dermal wound healing in young rats.

URL: https://pubmed.ncbi.nlm.nih.gov/20523108/

Authors: Nevin K. G.; T. Rajamojan

MY Summary: This is a primary study where Virgin Coconut Oil was tested on 18 rats - divided into 3 groups of 6 rats: a control group, a 0.5 ml treatment, and a 1 ml treatment - to evaluate its effect on minor skin wounds. The coconut oil did increase healing speed and "the beneficial effect of VCO [Virgin Coconut Oil] can be attributed to the cumulative effect of various biologically active minor components present in it."

Citation: Nevin KG, Rajamohan T. Effect of topical application of virgin coconut oil on skin components and antioxidant status during dermal wound healing in young rats. Skin Pharmacol Physiol. 2010;23(6):290-7. doi: 10.1159/000313516. Epub 2010 Jun 3. PMID: 20523108.

Title: Anti-Inflammatory and Skin Barrier Repair Effects of Topical Application of Some Plant Oils

URL: https://www.ncbi.nlm.nih.gov/pmc/articles/PMC5796020/

Authors: Tzu-Kai Lin; Lily Zhong; Juan Luis Santiago

MY Summary: This is a secondary/tertiary study on the beneficial effects of 19 oils, to include Olive oil, Coconut oil, and Avocado oil.

It first talks about the skin, including its function, structure, water-barrier, wound healing - including the 4 stages: "hemostasis, inflammation, proliferation, and tissue remodeling" - and aging. Then it provides detailed general information about oils, especially the composition and also the basic interactions and benefits of specific components of oils. Next, it summarizes the benefits and interactions of each specific oil of the 19 oils listed. "Topical applications of plant oils may have different effect on the skin according to their composition and the pathophysiological context [the 'how' or process of things working] of the skin." "When applied topically, constituents of plant oils [...] may act synergistically by several mechanisms: [...]"

Citation: Lin TK, Zhong L, Santiago JL. Anti-Inflammatory and Skin Barrier Repair Effects of Topical Application of Some Plant Oils. Int J Mol Sci. 2017 Dec 27;19(1):70. doi: 10.3390/ijms19010070. PMID: 29280987; PMCID: PMC5796020.

Title: In vitro anti-inflammatory and skin protective properties of Virgin coconut oil

URL: https://www.ncbi.nlm.nih.gov/pmc/articles/PMC6335493/

Authors: Sandeep R. Varma; Thiyagarajan O. Sivaprakasam; Ilavarasu Arumugam; N. Dilip; M. Raghuraman; K.B. Pavan; Mohammed Rafiq; Rangesh Paramesh

MY Summary: This is a primary study, in petri dishes. Virgin Coconut Oil reduced the production of 5 inflammatory cytokines, leading to a dramatic reduction in overall inflammation. Also, the Coconut oil augmented Involucrin, which is an essential and protective protein component in top-layer skin cells, Filaggrin, which binds skin cells together to create a strong, healthy, and unperturbed barrier, and Aquaporin, which facilitates water transportation, making it essential for skin moisturization.

Citation: Varma SR, Sivaprakasam TO, Arumugam I, Dilip N, Raghuraman M, Pavan KB, Rafiq M, Paramesh R. In vitro anti-inflammatory and skin protective properties of Virgin coconut oil. J Tradit Complement Med. 2018 Jan 17;9(1):5-14. doi: 10.1016/j.jtcme.2017.06.012. PMID: 30671361; PMCID: PMC6335493.

Title: Potential Effects of Phenolic Compounds That Can Be Found in Olive Oil on Wound Healing

URL: https://pubmed.ncbi.nlm.nih.gov/34359512/

Authors: Lucia Melguizo-Rodríguez; Elvira de Luna-Bertos; Javier Ramos-Torrecillas; Rebeca Illescas-Montesa; Victor Javier Costela-Ruiz; Olga García-Martínez

MY Summary: This is a secondary/tertiary study. "Results of in vitro and animal studies demonstrate that polyphenols [...] present in EVOO [Extra Virgin Olive Oil], participate in different aspects of wound healing, accelerating this process through their anti-inflammatory, antioxidant, and antimicrobial properties and their stimulation of angiogenic activities required for granulation tissue formation and wound re-epithelialization".

Citation: Melguizo-Rodríguez L, de Luna-Bertos E, Ramos-Torrecillas J, Illescas-Montesa R, Costela-Ruiz VJ, García-Martínez O. Potential Effects of Phenolic Compounds That Can Be Found in Olive Oil on Wound Healing. Foods. 2021 Jul 15;10(7):1642. doi: 10.3390/foods10071642. PMID: 34359512; PMCID: PMC8307686.

Title: The effect of topical olive oil on the healing of foot ulcer in patients with type 2 diabetes: a double-blind randomized clinical trial study in Iran

URL: https://www.ncbi.nlm.nih.gov/pmc/articles/PMC4428202/

Authors: Morteza Nasiri, Sadigheh Fayazi; Simin Jahani; Leila Yazdanpanah; Mohammad Hossein Haghighizadeh

MY Summary: This is a primary study: a clinical trial, lasting 4 weeks, containing one control group of 17 people obtaining a normal care routine and one intervention group of 17 people obtaining a normal care routine plus topical application of olive oil. This study observed how topical application of olive oil affected the healing of diabetic foot ulcers. Olive oil greatly reduced ulcer area and depth, though drainage was unaffected, and complete ulcer healing was 13.3% in the control group vs 73.3% in the intervention group; "also, there were no adverse effects to report during the study in [the] intervention group."

Citation: Nasiri M, Fayazi S, Jahani S, Yazdanpanah L, Haghighizadeh MH. The effect of topical olive oil on the healing of foot ulcer in patients with type 2 diabetes: a double-blind randomized clinical trial study in Iran. J Diabetes Metab Disord. 2015 Apr 29;14:38. doi: 10.1186/s40200-015-0167-9. PMID: 25969821; PMCID: PMC4428202.

Title: Anti-Inflammatory and Restorative Effects of Olives in Topical Application

URL: https://www.ncbi.nlm.nih.gov/pmc/articles/PMC8257351/

Authors: Mahdiyeh Taheri; Leila Amiri-Farahani

MY Summary: This is a secondary study. The first section is a great synopsis of the article. Then it gives a brief summary of the reason for looking into this. After going over the process of primary research paper selection, it states the composition of olive oil and gives a few sentences to state how it helps the healing process generally. Next, it summarizes the information on the subjects of several of the studies, to include treatment for nipple sores, pressure ulcers, chronic ulcers, diabetic foot ulcers, perineal ulcers, diaper rash, and eczema. Last, it gives the authors' conclusions.

Citation: Taheri M, Amiri-Farahani L. Anti-Inflammatory and Restorative Effects of Olives in Topical Application. Dermatol Res Pract. 2021 Jun 26;2021:9927976. doi: 10.1155/2021/9927976. PMID: 34257643; PMCID: PMC8257351.

Title: Potential Effects of Phenolic Compounds That Can Be Found in Olive Oil on Wound Healing

URL: https://www.ncbi.nlm.nih.gov/pmc/articles/PMC8307686/

Authors: Lucia Melguizo-Rodríguez; Elvira de Luna-Bertos; Javier Ramos-Torrecillas; Rebeca Illescas-Montesa; Victor Javier Costela-Ruiz; Olga García-Martínez

MY Summary: Most of this tertiary research paper goes over the individual components of olive oil and explains how they actually improve healing, including several specific findings from various primary studies.

Citation: Melguizo-Rodríguez L, de Luna-Bertos E, Ramos-Torrecillas J, Illescas-Montesa R, Costela-Ruiz VJ, García-Martínez O. Potential Effects of Phenolic Compounds That Can Be Found in Olive Oil on Wound Healing. Foods. 2021 Jul 15;10(7):1642. doi: 10.3390/foods10071642. PMID: 34359512; PMCID: PMC8307686.

Title: Effect of Semisolid Formulation of Persea Americana Mill (Avocado) Oil on Wound Healing in Rats

URL: https://www.ncbi.nlm.nih.gov/pmc/articles/PMC3614059/

Authors: Ana Paula de Oliveira; Eryvelton de Souza Franco; Rafaella Rodrigues Barreto; Daniele Pires Cordeiro; Rebeca Gonçalves de Melo; Camila Maria Ferreira de Aquino; Antonio Alfredo Rodrigues e Silva; Paloma Lys de Medeiros; Teresinha Gonçalves da Silva; Alexandre José da Silva Góes; and Maria Bernadete de Sousa Maia

MY Summary: After the initial summary, it quickly explains pertinent information relating to the process of wound healing, how various (but specific) fatty acids impact the process, and the fatty acid and vitamin profile of avocado oil; all of this details why this primary study - an animal study - was done and the reason for the 4 different options of topical application: Semisolid formulation of avocado (SSFAO - essentially super-mashed avocado pulp), an oil rich in essential fatty acids (EFA - essentially the avocado minus everything that isn't fatty acids), avocado oil (like bought at a store), and petroleum jelly. Petroleum jelly was the 1st control; ordinary avocado oil was the 2nd control / 1st experimental; SSFAO was the 1st modified experimental; EFA was the 2nd modified experimental; if pictured, imagine a capital "Y", where the writing line that the "Y" is on top of is no treatment/normal healing, the bottom point on the "Y" is petroleum jelly, the middle point on the "Y" is ordinary avocado oil, and the two high points on the "Y" are the SSFAO (more whole avocado style and least refined) and the EFA (more active ingredient style and most refined). Results: SSFAO, EFA, and Avocado oil improved healing compared to control (petroleum jelly). It appears to me that EFA resulted in the most physical regeneration material, but

SSFAO resulted in the least inflammation and best structure repair, while Avocado oil was the blend of the two.

I add that I believe it should be noted that they used Petroleum Jelly as a control, but the healing rate from Petroleum Jelly application is still greater than no material application, such as by simply putting on a bandage and keeping the wound dry. As such, although the Avocado oil and its modified forms SSFAO and EFA were more effective than Petroleum Jelly, it does not reveal the complete extent of increased healing provided when nothing is applied.

Citation: de Oliveira AP, Franco Ede S, Rodrigues Barreto R, Cordeiro DP, de Melo RG, de Aquino CM, E Silva AA, de Medeiros PL, da Silva TG, Góes AJ, Maia MB. Effect of semisolid formulation of persea americana mill (avocado) oil on wound healing in rats. Evid Based Complement Alternat Med. 2013;2013:472382. doi: 10.1155/2013/472382. Epub 2013 Mar 19. PMID: 23573130; PMCID: PMC3614059.

Title: Protective Mechanisms of Avocado Oil Extract Against Ototoxicity

URL: https://www.ncbi.nlm.nih.gov/pmc/articles/PMC7230542/

Authors: Thu Nguyen Minh Pham; Seo Yeon Jeong; Do Hoon Kim; Yu Hwa Park; Jung Suk Lee; Kye Wan Lee; In Seok Moon; Se Young Choung; Seung Hyun Kim; Tong Ho Kang; Kwang Won Jeong

MY Summary: This was a primary study, a study with petri dishes, and the main purpose of this study was not to determine if Avocado oil could reduce drug-caused damage to hearing, especially to the small hairs involved in the perception of sound. In this study, a few things were confirmed. 1st, the primary cause of damage, and the resultant cell death, from aminoglycoside antibiotics (such as gentamicin, amikacin, tobramycin, neomycin, and streptomycin) is free radical production. 2nd, Avocado oil directly scavenges free radicals, which immediately prevents damage caused by them. 3rd, Avocado oil stimulates cellular detoxification and increases Glutathione levels. 4th, Avocado oil reduces cellular production of inflammatory cytokines, which results in lower inflammation and tempering immune cell activity.

In a nutshell, Avocado oil reduces inflammation, reduces damage from overactivity of the immune system in the immediate region of application, and protects cells from damage and death by cellular toxins (prolonging cell survival which increases cellular proliferation resulting in faster tissue regeneration).

Citation: Pham TNM, Jeong SY, Kim DH, Park YH, Lee JS, Lee KW, Moon IS, Choung SY, Kim SH, Kang TH, Jeong KW. Protective Mechanisms of Avocado Oil Extract Against Ototoxicity. Nutrients. 2020 Mar 29;12(4):947. doi: 10.3390/nu12040947. PMID: 32235401; PMCID: PMC7230542.

Title: The Role of Vitamin A in Wound Healing

URL: https://pubmed.ncbi.nlm.nih.gov/31389093/

Authors: Monica E Polcz; Adrian Barbul

MY Summary: Vitamin A is a primary regulator of cellular reproduction, which means increased vitamin A also increases cell reproduction, increasing tissue repair, and vitamin A deficiency leads to slow healing. Also, Vitamin A is antiinflammatory.

Citation: Polcz ME, Barbul A. The Role of Vitamin A in Wound Healing. Nutr Clin Pract. 2019 Oct;34(5):695-700. doi: 10.1002/ncp.10376. Epub 2019 Aug 7. PMID: 31389093.

Title: Supplemental vitamin A prevents the tumor-induced defect in wound healing

URL: https://pubmed.ncbi.nlm.nih.gov/2310237/

Authors: J Weinzweig; S M Levenson; G Rettura; N Weinzweig; J Mendecki; T H Chang; E Seifter

MY Summary: This is a primary study - an animal study. Tumors impair the quality of skin healing. Vitamin A supplementation mostly negated the impairment of the tumors. For example: If the tumors reduced the healing ability from 10 points to 5 points, then Vitamin A would increase it to 9 points, eliminating the tumor but not giving vit A would be 7 points, and eliminating the tumors in addition to vit a supplementation would be 9 points. Vitamin A nor the removal of the tumors completely negated the healing impairment of the tumors, but in such cases, vit A did better than the removal of the tumors, though it was not synergistic with the removal of the tumors as it only went to the extent that it would have gone without the removal.

Citation: Weinzweig J, Levenson SM, Rettura G, Weinzweig N, Mendecki J, Chang TH, Seifter E. Supplemental vitamin A prevents the tumor-induced defect in wound healing. Ann Surg. 1990 Mar;211(3):269-76. PMID: 2310237; PMCID: PMC1358431.

Title: Vitamin C and human wound healing

URL: https://pubmed.ncbi.nlm.nih.gov/7038579/

Authors: W M Ringsdorf Jr; E Cheraskin

MY Summary: Basic summary of a primary study - some clinical trials. Doctors in this study gave post-surgery patients up to 50 times (5,000%) the recommended daily dose of vitamin C part-way through the healing process. They discovered that the extra vitamin C caused new skin growth to be much better than the pre-extra-vitamin-C skin, but it did not change the previously formed skin to become the same superior quality as the post-extra-vitamin-C skin.

Citation: Ringsdorf WM Jr, Cheraskin E. Vitamin C and human wound healing. Oral Surg Oral Med Oral Pathol. 1982 Mar;53(3):231-6. doi: 10.1016/0030-4220(82)90295-x. PMID: 7038579.

Title: The Review on Properties of Aloe Vera in Healing of Cutaneous Wounds

URL: https://www.ncbi.nlm.nih.gov/pmc/articles/PMC4452276/

Authors: Seyyed Abbas Hashemi; Seyyed Abdollah Madani; Saied Abediankenari

MY Summary: "aloe vera improves the wound healing as well as other procedures both clinically and experimentally". The first few sections go into some detail about various factors of wound healing generally. Then it gives some information on aloe vera, to include its component analysis. Next, it goes into segmental explanations of how Aloe Vera benefits the healing process. In the first segmental explanation, it tells of a significantly active compound known as glucomannan, which increases activation of growth factors. Then it gives a brief explanation of growth factors and their essential effects.

Citation: Hashemi SA, Madani SA, Abediankenari S. The Review on Properties of Aloe Vera in Healing of Cutaneous Wounds. Biomed Res Int. 2015;2015:714216. doi: 10.1155/2015/714216. Epub 2015 May 19. PMID: 26090436; PMCID: PMC4452276.

Title: Pharmacological Update Properties of Aloe Vera and its Major Active Constituents

URL: https://www.ncbi.nlm.nih.gov/pmc/articles/PMC7144722/

Authors: Marta Sánchez; Elena González-Burgos; Irene Iglesias; M. Pilar Gómez-Serranillos

MY Summary: This is a secondary study of the benefits of Aloe Vera, especially in the mechanisms of action (the how/process of what something accomplishes). First it gives a synopsis of Aloe Vera, and then it gives a list of studies in a very bare-bone manner: Aloe Vera product, the application subject, and the primary results/findings. Next, it summarized the findings for the benefits of the digestive system, such as with mouth conditions, mucus secretions, indigestion, etc. In section 3 it discusses various benefits for the skin, including with wound healing, to include: "clinical trials have demonstrated that Aloe vera facilitated rapid tissue epithelialization and granulation in burns, promoted healing of cesarean wound, and accelerated wound healing of split-thickness skin graft donor sites" - clinical trials (experimental treatment group vs normal treatment group test concerning humans) have shown that Aloe Vera enhanced the skin's ability to regrow new outer-layer (and protective) skin and new capillaries, enhanced healing of a surgical cut, and enhanced healing of spots where skin was removed to be used on other parts of the body. The next sections covered: anti-inflammatory action, anti-cancer effects, anti-diabetic effects, antioxidant properties, bone modulation, beneficial effects on the heart and blood, and its antimicrobial effects. The last statement in the conclusion states "The promising results of basic research encourage a greater number of clinical trials to test the clinical application of Aloe vera and its main compounds, particularly on bone protection, cancer, and diabetes.".

Citation: Sánchez M, González-Burgos E, Iglesias I, Gómez-Serranillos MP. Pharmacological Update Properties of Aloe Vera and its Major Active Constituents. Molecules. 2020 Mar 13;25(6):1324. doi: 10.3390/molecules25061324. PMID: 32183224; PMCID: PMC7144722.

Title: Effects of petrolatum on stratum corneum structure and function

URL: https://pubmed.ncbi.nlm.nih.gov/1564142/

Authors: R Ghadially; L Halkier-Sorensen; P M Elias

MY Summary: Vaseline Petroleum Jelly, after application to the skin, occupies intercellular spaces; by doing so it reduces water loss from the skin while also accelerating the skin's water barrier recovery.

Citation: Ghadially R, Halkier-Sorensen L, Elias PM. Effects of petrolatum on stratum corneum structure and function. J Am Acad Dermatol. 1992 Mar;26(3 Pt 2):387-96. doi: 10.1016/0190-9622(92)70060-s. PMID: 1564142.

Title: Petrolatum: Barrier repair and antimicrobial responses underlying this "inert" moisturizer

URL: https://pubmed.ncbi.nlm.nih.gov/26431582/

Authors: Tali Czarnowicki; Dana Malajian; Saakshi Khattri; Joel Correa da Rosa; Riana Dutt; Robert Finney; Nikhil Dhingra; Peng Xiangyu; Hui Xu; Yeriel D Estrada; Xiuzhong Zheng; Patricia Gilleaudeau; Mary Sullivan-Whalen; Mayte Suaréz-Fariñas; Avner Shemer; James G Krueger; Emma Guttman-Yassky

MY Summary: This is a primary study, a clinical trial. "Conclusions: Petrolatum robustly modulates antimicrobials and epidermal differentiation barrier measures. These data shed light on the beneficial molecular responses of petrolatum in barrier-defective states, such as AD [Atopic Dermatitis] and postoperative wound care."

Citation: Czarnowicki T, Malajian D, Khattri S, Correa da Rosa J, Dutt R, Finney R, Dhingra N, Xiangyu P, Xu H, Estrada YD, Zheng X, Gilleaudeau P, Sullivan-Whalen M, Suaréz-Fariñas M, Shemer A, Krueger JG, Guttman-Yassky E. Petrolatum: Barrier repair and antimicrobial responses underlying this "inert" moisturizer. J Allergy Clin Immunol. 2016 Apr;137(4):1091-1102.e7. doi: 10.1016/j.jaci.2015.08.013. Epub 2015 Oct 1. PMID: 26431582.

Title: Postoperative wound care after dermatologic procedures: a comparison of 2 commonly used petrolatum-based ointments

URL: https://pubmed.ncbi.nlm.nih.gov/23377388/

Authors: Adisbeth Morales-Burgos; Michael P Loosemore; Leonard H Goldberg

MY Summary: White petroleum jelly can be used to keep wounds moist to the proper extent. This is simply a 1 paragraph abstract....

Citation: Morales-Burgos A, Loosemore MP, Goldberg LH. Postoperative wound care after dermatologic procedures: a comparison of 2 commonly used petrolatum-based ointments. J Drugs Dermatol. 2013 Feb;12(2):163-4. PMID: 23377388.

Title: Wound Healing and Anti-Inflammatory Effect in Animal Models of Calendula officinalis L. Growing in Brazil

URL: https://www.ncbi.nlm.nih.gov/pmc/articles/PMC3270572/

Authors: Leila Maria Leal Parente; Ruy de Souza Lino Júnior; Leonice Manrique Faustino Tresvenzol; Marina Clare Vinaud; José Realino de Paula; Neusa Margarida Paulo

MY Summary: "Calendula officinalis growing in Brazil presented anti-inflammatory and antibacterial activities as well as the capability of stimulating fibroplasia and angiogenesis. Therefore, the C. officinalis extracts act in a positive form on the inflammatory and proliferative phases of the healing process of cutaneous wounds." Calendula's scientific name is Calendula Officinalis. Fibroplasia is new tissue, and is pink if healthy or red and bleedy if unhealthy.

Citation: Parente LM, Lino Júnior Rde S, Tresvenzol LM, Vinaud MC, de Paula JR, Paulo NM. Wound Healing and Anti-Inflammatory Effect in Animal Models of Calendula officinalis L. Growing in Brazil. Evid Based Complement Alternat Med. 2012;2012:375671. doi: 10.1155/2012/375671. Epub 2012 Jan 24. PMID: 22315631; PMCID: PMC3270572.

Title: Use of calendula ointment after episiotomy: a randomized clinical trial

URL: https://pubmed.ncbi.nlm.nih.gov/32460565/

Authors: Carlo De Angelis; Arianna Di Stadio; Silvia Vitale; Gabriele Saccone; Maria Chiara De Angelis; Brunella Zizolfi; Attilio Di Spiezio Sardo

MY Summary: This is a primary study, a clinical trial, involving the recovery of minor surgery (episiotomy) to reduce the extent of harm and risk in a difficult 'natural' childbirth, and compared normal treatment to normal treatment plus calendula ointment. "Results:

During the study, 100 women agreed to take part in the study, underwent randomization, and were enrolled in this trial. Of the 100 randomized women, 50 were randomized to the calendula ointment group, and 50 to the control group. No women were excluded after randomization or lost to follow up. Women who received calendula ointment after episiotomy compared to standard care had a significantly lower pain level starting from day two and during all the follow-up. Calendula ointment also improve wound healing in terms of redness and edema."

Citation: De Angelis C, Di Stadio A, Vitale S, Saccone G, Angelis MC, Zizolfi B, Di Spiezio Sardo A. Use of calendula ointment after episiotomy: a randomized clinical trial. J Matern Fetal Neonatal Med. 2022 May;35(10):1860-1864. doi: 10.1080/14767058.2020.1770219. Epub 2020 May 27. PMID: 32460565.

Title: Treatment of acute wounds in hand with Calendula officinalis L.: A randomized trial

URL: https://pubmed.ncbi.nlm.nih.gov/34674610/

Authors: Giana Silveira Giostri; Eduardo Murilo Novak; Marcelo Buzzi; Luiz Cesar Guarita-Souza

MY Summary: This was a primary study, a clinical trial, comparing the treatment of minor wounds on the hands with mineral oil (20 people) versus calendula (20 people). "healing [...] acute wounds of the hand and fingers with [Calendula] led to a faster epithelization". The healing in the calendula group was about 1.5 times faster than in the mineral oil group: epithelization in the calendula group averaged 9.5% per day but only averaged 6.2% per day in the mineral oil group.

Citation: Giostri GS, Novak EM, Buzzi M, Guarita-Souza LC. Treatment of acute wounds in hand with Calendula officinalis L.: A randomized trial. Tissue Barriers. 2022 Jul 3;10(3):1994822. doi: 10.1080/21688370.2021.1994822. Epub 2021 Oct 21. Erratum in: Tissue Barriers. 2022 Apr 7;:2056359. PMID: 34674610; PMCID: PMC9359387.

Title: Phytochemistry and Biological Activity of Medicinal Plants in Wound Healing: An Overview of Current Research

URL: https://www.ncbi.nlm.nih.gov/pmc/articles/PMC9182061/

Authors: Stefania Vitale; Sara Colanero; Martina Placidi; Giovanna Di Emidio; Carla Tatone; Fernanda Amicarelli; and Anna Maria D'Alessandro

MY Summary: This is a tertiary study on wound healing in general. Following its summary (the "abstract"), it first delves into a moderate and somewhat detailed explanation into wound healing itself, to include details and reasons for the 4 steps of the wound healing process. Then it very briefly talks about the basics of wound dressings. Next, it goes into mild detail of a variety of herbal applications, including Yarrow, <u>Aloe Vera</u>, Chinese ground orchid, <u>Calendula</u>, Casearia Sylvestris, Saffron, Turmeric, Licorice, common Mallow, Plantago, Sage, and Rosemary. <u>Some key notes in the conclusion</u>: "Effective treatment of wounds depends upon the interaction of appropriate cell types, cell surface receptors, and the extracellular matrix with the therapeutic agents. Due to the complexity of skin tissue structure, the development of an ideal medication, which can lead to a rapid and effective healing process, remains a challenge." <u>and</u> "There has been an increasing interest in the synergistic effect of different extracts with specific phytocomponents. For example, when B. striata's extract polysaccharides, primarily glucomannans, are enriched with B. striata extract mainly containing polyphenols, more effective healing of wounds is observed" and "different therapeutic strategies should be used simultaneously in the management of wounds, especially chronic wounds, to accelerate the wound-healing process and avoid wound complications."

Citation: Vitale S, Colanero S, Placidi M, Di Emidio G, Tatone C, Amicarelli F, D'Alessandro AM. Phytochemistry and Biological Activity of Medicinal Plants in Wound Healing: An Overview of Current Research. Molecules. 2022 Jun 1;27(11):3566. doi: 10.3390/molecules27113566. PMID: 35684503; PMCID: PMC9182061.

Title: Extracts of Eucalyptus alba Promote Diabetic Wound Healing by Inhibiting α-Glucosidase and Stimulating Cell Proliferation

URL: https://www.ncbi.nlm.nih.gov/pmc/articles/PMC9033357/

Authors: Rabia Mumtaz; Muhammad Zubair; Muhammad Asaf Khan; Saima Muzammil; Muhammad Hussnain Siddique

MY Summary: The section "Conclusion" states: "Eucalyptus alba leaves dried at 10°C, 30°C, 50°C, and 100°C extracted in different solvents (ethanol, methanol, and acetone) were investigated for diabetic wound healing activity. Findings of the current study revealed that extracts of E. alba effectively stimulated the in vitro cell proliferation. The antioxidant and antidiabetic activities of the extracts have also supported the diabetic wound healing potential of E. alba leaf extracts. Furthermore, the plant extracts inhibited the growth of hepatocellular carcinoma [type of skin cancer] (Huh-7) cell line but showed no signs of cytotoxicity on retinal pigment epithelial (RPE) cells. Overall, best results were obtained with leaves dried at 10°C and extracted in ethanol" [I, Peter, did the underlining]. The study suggests that E. alba leaves might be a potential natural source for diabetic wound healing.".

Citation: Mumtaz R, Zubair M, Khan MA, Muzammil S, Siddique MH. Extracts of Eucalyptus alba Promote Diabetic Wound Healing by Inhibiting α-Glucosidase and Stimulating Cell Proliferation. Evid Based Complement Alternat Med. 2022 Apr 15;2022:4953105. doi: 10.1155/2022/4953105. PMID: 35463094; PMCID: PMC9033357.

Title: Essential oil-loaded lipid nanoparticles for wound healing

URL: https://pubmed.ncbi.nlm.nih.gov/29343956/

Authors: Francesca Saporito; Giuseppina Sandri; Maria Cristina Bonferoni; Silvia Rossi; Cinzia Boselli; Antonia Icaro Cornaglia; Barbara Mannucci; Pietro Grisoli; Barbara Vigani; Franca Ferrari

MY Summary: This was a summary of an animal study. "NLC [Nano-structured Lipid Carriers] based on olive oil and loaded with eucalyptus oil showed appropriate physical-chemical properties, good bioadhesion, cytocompatibility, in vitro proliferation enhancement, and wound healing properties toward fibroblasts, associated to antimicrobial properties. Moreover, the in vivo results evidenced the capability of these NLC to enhance the healing process. Olive oil, which is characterized by a high content of oleic acid, proved to exert a synergic effect with eucalyptus oil with respect to antimicrobial activity and wound repair promotion."

Citation: Saporito F, Sandri G, Bonferoni MC, Rossi S, Boselli C, Icaro Cornaglia A, Mannucci B, Grisoli P, Vigani B, Ferrari F. Essential oil-loaded lipid nanoparticles for wound healing. Int J Nanomedicine. 2017 Dec 27;13:175-186. doi: 10.2147/IJN.S152529. PMID: 29343956; PMCID: PMC5747963.

Title: Eucalyptus oleosa Essential Oils: Chemical Composition and Antimicrobial and Antioxidant Activities of the Oils from Different Plant Parts (Stems, Leaves, Flowers and Fruits)

URL: https://www.ncbi.nlm.nih.gov/pmc/articles/PMC6259913/

Authors: Hajer Naceur Ben Marzoug; Mehrez Romdhane; Ahmed Lebrihi; Florence Mathieu; François Couderc; Manef Abderraba; Mohamed Larbi Khouja; Jalloul Bouajila

MY Summary: "the essential oils of Eucalyptus species possesses important biological activities including diaphoretic [cause to sweat], disinfectant [antimicrobial], antimalarial [helps treat and prevent malaria], antiseptic [prevents microbial growth], analgesic [pain relieving], antiinflammatory, antibacterial, expectorant [clears mucus], and antioxidant properties". After the introduction to some aspects of Eucalyptus, it gives a component breakdown of the oil. Next it states their findings on the antioxidant activity, which is moderately good, followed by some antimicrobial activity. After the antimicrobial activity, they detailed how they conducted their experiments and ended with their brief conclusion.

The oils from the different parts of the plant were tested against 7 bacteria (b) and 5 fungi (f). The average and range of MIC (Minimum Inhibitory Concentration - think the smallest concentration to give any antiseptic activity, however small) for the oils from all parts of the plants are: (b) **Hay bacillus**: Average: 0.288%, Best: Immature flowers - 0.093%, Worst: Adult leaves - 0.465%; (b) **Staphylococcus aureus**: Average: 0.202%, Best: Adult leaves/Immature flowers - 0.186%, Worst: Fruits - 0.240%; (b) **Listeria monocytogenes**: Average: 0.202%, Best: Adult leaves/Immature flowers - 0.186%, Worst: Fruits - 0.240%; (b) **Pseudomonas aeruginosa**: Average: 0.455%, Best: Immature flowers - 0.279%, Worst: Adult leaves -

0.651%; (b) **Salmonella enterica**: Average: 0.269%, Best: Immature flowers - 0.186%, Worst: Fruits - 0.320%; (b) **Escherichia coli**: Average: 0.245%, Best: Immature flowers - 0.186%, Worst: Fruits - 0.320%; (b) **Klebsiella pneumoniae**: Average: 0.296%, Best: Immature flowers - 0.186%, Worst: Adult leaves - 0.465%; (f) **Saccharomyces cerevisiae (brewer's yeast)**: Average: 0.339%, Best: Immature flowers - 0.279%, Worst: Adult leaves - 0.465%; (f) **Candida albicans**: Average: 0.359%, Best: Immature flowers - 0.279%, Worst: Adult leaves - 0.465%; (f) **Aspergillus ochraceus**: Average: 0.433%, Best: Immature flowers - 0.279%, Worst: Fruits - 0.600%; (f) **Mucor ramamnianus**: Average: 0.480%, Best: Immature flowers - 0.279%, Worst: Adult leaves - 0.651%; (f) **Fusarium culmorum**: Average: 0.386%, Best: Fruits - 0.320%, Worst: Adult leaves - 0.465%.

Citation: Ben Marzoug HN, Romdhane M, Lebrihi A, Mathieu F, Couderc F, Abderraba M, Khouja ML, Bouajila J. Eucalyptus oleosa essential oils: chemical composition and antimicrobial and antioxidant activities of the oils from different plant parts (stems, leaves, flowers and fruits). Molecules. 2011 Feb 17;16(2):1695-709. doi: 10.3390/molecules16021695. PMID: 21330958; PMCID: PMC6259913.

Title: Chemical Composition, Antioxidant, Antimicrobial, and Phytotoxic Potential of Eucalyptus grandis × E. urophylla Leaves Essential Oils

URL: https://www.ncbi.nlm.nih.gov/pmc/articles/PMC7962113/

Authors: Lijun Zhou; Jiajia Li; Qingbo Kong; Siyuan Luo; Jie Wang; Shiling Feng; Ming Yuan; Tao Chen; Shu Yuan; Chunbang Ding

MY Summary: These are the results of a tested hybrid of two species of Eucalyptus trees. In the component breakdown, and of great significance, one of the ordinarily major components - Eucalyptol - is found in a dramatically smaller degree. Despite this change, alternate components to Eucalyptol, also produced by the precursors to Eucalyptol, still resulted in decent antioxidant ability and strong antimicrobial activity. MICs (Minimum Inhibitory Concentrations) for 6 bacteria were: Escherichia coli 0.0091%, Hay bacillus 0.0091%, Pseudomonas aeruginosa 0.0023%, Staphylococcus aureus 0.0045%, Salmonella typhimurium 0.0023%, Bacillus cereus 0.0045%. The minimum concentration for 100% inhibition of 6 fungi were: Trichoderma longibrachiatum 2%, Botrytis cinerea 1%, Colletotrichum acutatum 2%, Colletotrichum gloeosporioides 1%, Fusarium oxysporum 2%, Fusarium graminearum 4%.

Citation: Zhou L, Li J, Kong Q, Luo S, Wang J, Feng S, Yuan M, Chen T, Yuan S, Ding C. Chemical Composition, Antioxidant, Antimicrobial, and Phytotoxic Potential of Eucalyptus grandis × E. urophylla Leaves Essential Oils. Molecules. 2021 Mar 7;26(5):1450. doi: 10.3390/molecules26051450. PMID: 33800071; PMCID: PMC7962113.

Title: Appraisal on the wound healing potential of Melaleuca alternifolia and Rosmarinus officinalis L. essential oil-loaded chitosan topical preparations

URL: https://www.ncbi.nlm.nih.gov/pmc/articles/PMC6746351/

Authors: Rola M. Labib (Supervision, Writing – review & editing); Iriny M. Ayoub (Supervision, Writing – review & editing); Haidy E. Michel (Methodology); Mina Mehanny (Methodology); Verena Kamil (Investigation); Meryl Hany (Investigation); Mirette Magdy

(Investigation); Aya Moataz (Investigation); Boula Maged (Investigation); Ahmed Mohamed (Investigation)

MY Summary: This is a primary study, an animal study, comparing 6 healing methods to compare wound contraction speeds. This paper also breaks down the components of both Tea Tree and Rosemary oils. "[Tea Tree Oil] was officially identified as an antiseptic in 1923 by Dr. Arthur Penfold who reported that tea tree oil was 11 times stronger in activity than phenol, the standard antiseptic at that time. This "magic healing oil" was supplied to the Australian army during World War II as it was the best possible available treatment against infection from cuts, wounds and bites". Although I will not add the super useful pictures and actual table provided, one key table of information is as follows (rounded amounts), where 100% means completely contracted by that day:

Day 7: Nothing applied to wound contracted 20%, Nolaver applied to wound contracted 35%, Chitosan applied to wound contracted 25%, Chitosan with Tea Tree applied to wound contracted 45%, Chitosan with Rosemary applied to wound contracted 45%, Chitosan with Tea Tree and Rosemary applied to wound contracted 55%. Day 14: Nothing applied to wound contracted 40%, Nolaver applied to wound contracted 80%, Chitosan applied to wound contracted 55%, Chitosan with Tea Tree applied to wound contracted 80%, Chitosan with Rosemary applied to wound contracted 70%, Chitosan with Tea Tree and Rosemary applied to wound contracted 90%.

Citation: Labib RM, Ayoub IM, Michel HE, Mehanny M, Kamil V, Hany M, Magdy M, Moataz A, Maged B, Mohamed A. Appraisal on the wound healing potential of Melaleuca alternifolia and Rosmarinus officinalis L. essential oil-loaded chitosan topical preparations. PLoS One. 2019 Sep 16;14(9):e0219561. doi:

10.1371/journal.pone.0219561. PMID: 31525200; PMCID: PMC6746351.

Title: In vitro antimicrobial effect of essential tea tree oil(Melaleuca alternifolia), thymol, and carvacrol on microorganisms isolated from cases of bovine clinical mastitis

URL: https://www.ncbi.nlm.nih.gov/pmc/articles/PMC9543160/

Authors: Lysett Corona-Gómez; Laura Hernández-Andrade; Susana Mendoza-Elvira; Feliciano Milián Suazo; Daniel Israel Ricardo-González; David Quintanar-Guerrero

MY Summary: This study particularly involves bacterial infections taken from cattle, but these same bacteria also cause human infections. In this study they include their process and the specifics of the experiments. In the conclusion it states: "The in vitro bactericidal activity of Melaleuca alternifolia tea tree oil (TTO), thymol, and carvacrol against field isolates and ATCC strains of Staphylococcus spp, Streptococcus spp, Escherichia coli, Klebsiella pneumoniae, and Candida albicans isolated from clinical mastitis were evaluated. Of the natural oils tested, thymol had the largest inhibition halo diameter for most of these strains. The combinations of thymol+carvacrol and TTO+thymol showed additive activity with the group of gram-negative bacteria and C. albicans. In vitro testing of natural active ingredients has revealed inhibition rates above 70% compared to positive controls. This indicates that the combinations of thymol+carvacrol and TTO+thymol can be used to develop formulations as alternatives to conventional antimicrobial therapy for bovine mastitis, or to improve the efficacy of existing treatments."

Citation: Corona-Gómez L, Hernández-Andrade L, Mendoza-Elvira S, Suazo FM, Ricardo-González DI, Quintanar-Guerrero D. In vitro antimicrobial effect of essential tea tree oil(Melaleuca alternifolia), thymol, and carvacrol on microorganisms isolated from cases of bovine clinical mastitis. Int J Vet Sci Med. 2022 Sep 29;10(1):72-79. doi: 10.1080/23144599.2022.2123082. PMID: 36259046; PMCID: PMC9543160.

Title: Physical and Antibacterial Properties of Peppermint Essential Oil Loaded Poly (ε-caprolactone) (PCL) Electrospun Fiber Mats for Wound Healing

URL: https://www.ncbi.nlm.nih.gov/pmc/articles/PMC6988806/

Authors: Irem Unalan; Benedikt Slavik; Andrea Buettner; Wolfgang H. Goldmann; Gerhard Frank; Aldo R. Boccaccini

MY Summary: This paper begins by explaining why they are doing this study of essential oil infused electrospun fiber mats (for injury healing purposes), to include how the EOs affect bacterial growth in applied areas. After explaining the details of the process of their experiment, they give the results, beginning with the effect peppermint EO had on the fibers of the electrospun fiber mats. "The antibacterial activity of PCL, PCLPEP1.5, PCLPEP3, and PCLPEP6 electrospun fiber mats was tested with Staphylococcus aureus as gram-positive bacteria and Escherichia coli as gram-negative bacteria, separately. As presented in Figure 8, the relative bacterial viability of samples was investigated at 3, 6, 24, and 48 h. During the 48 h incubation, PCLPEP1.5, PCLPEP3, and PCLPEP6 exhibited decreased bacterial viability compared to PCL electrospun fiber mats. Additionally, the antibacterial activity was enhanced with an increase of PEP concentration in PCLPEP1.5, PCLPEP3, and PCLPEP6. The PCLPEP6 composition showed the lowest bacterial viability (S. aureus; $50 \pm 3\%$ and E. coli; $70 \pm 2\%$) at 24 h incubation." PCL means just the electrospun fiber mat, PCLPEP1.5 means fiber mat with 1.5%

peppermint EO concentration; PCLPEP3 means fiber mat with 3% peppermint EO, and PCLPEP6 means fiber mat with 6% peppermint EO. Bacterial viability means the ability for the bacteria to survive - the lower the viability the stronger the antibacterial effect.

Citation: Unalan I, Slavik B, Buettner A, Goldmann WH, Frank G, Boccaccini AR. Physical and Antibacterial Properties of Peppermint Essential Oil Loaded Poly (ε-caprolactone) (PCL) Electrospun Fiber Mats for Wound Healing. Front Bioeng Biotechnol. 2019 Nov 26;7:346. doi: 10.3389/fbioe.2019.00346. PMID: 32039166; PMCID: PMC6988806.

Title: The Use of Menthol in Skin Wound Healing—Anti-Inflammatory Potential, Antioxidant Defense System Stimulation and Increased Epithelialization

URL: https://www.ncbi.nlm.nih.gov/pmc/articles/PMC8620938/

Authors: Ariane Leite Rozza; Fernando Pereira Beserra; Ana Júlia Vieira; Eduardo Oliveira de Souza; Carlos Alberto Hussni; Emanuel Ricardo Monteiro Martinez; Rafael Henrique Nóbrega; and Cláudia Helena Pellizzon

MY Summary: The abstract does a spectacular job at summarizing this paper.

"Wound healing involves inflammatory, proliferative, and remodeling phases, in which various cells and chemical intermediates are involved. This study aimed to investigate the skin wound healing potential of menthol, as well as the mechanisms involved in its effect, after 3, 7, or 14 days of treatment, according to the phases of wound healing. Skin wound was performed in the back of Wistar rats, which were topically treated with vehicle cream; collagenase-based cream (1.2 U/g); or menthol-based cream at 0.25%, 0.5%, or 1.0% over 3, 7, or 14 days. Menthol cream at 0.5% accelerated the healing right from the inflammatory phase (3 days) by decreasing mRNA expression of inflammatory cytokines TNF-α and Il-6. At the proliferative phase (7 days), menthol 0.5% increased the activity of antioxidant enzymes SOD, GR, and GPx, as well as the level of GSH, in addition to decreasing the levels of inflammatory cytokines TNF-α, IL-6, and IL-1β and augmenting mRNA expression for Ki-67, a marker of cellular proliferation. At the remodeling phase (14 days), levels of inflammatory cytokines were decreased, and the level of Il-10 and its mRNA expression were increased in the menthol 0.5% group. Menthol presented skin wound healing activity by modulating the antioxidant system of the cells and the inflammatory response, in addition to stimulating epithelialization."

All menthol extracts did better than the vehicle cream, and so did the collagenase-based cream; the menthol extracts did better than the collagenase-based cream until between 7 and 14 days, and as of day 14 the collagenase-based cream very slightly outperformed menthol cream at 0.25% and 1%, but not at 0.5%. Menthol cream at 0.5% performed the best out of all of the creams at every day of measurement.

Citation: Rozza AL, Beserra FP, Vieira AJ, Oliveira de Souza E, Hussni CA, Martinez ERM, Nóbrega RH, Pellizzon CH. The Use of Menthol in Skin Wound Healing-Anti-Inflammatory Potential, Antioxidant Defense System Stimulation and Increased Epithelialization. Pharmaceutics. 2021 Nov 9;13(11):1902. doi: 10.3390/pharmaceutics13111902. PMID: 34834317; PMCID: PMC8620938.

Title: Microbicide activity of clove essential oil (Eugenia caryophyllata)

URL: https://www.ncbi.nlm.nih.gov/pmc/articles/PMC3769004/

Authors: L. Nuñez; M. D' Aquino

MY Summary: "The influence of clove essential oil concentration, temperature and organic matter, in the antimicrobial activity of clove essential oil, was studied in this paper, through the determination of bacterial death kinetics. Escherichia coli, Staphylococcus aureus and Pseudomonas aeruginosa were the microorganisms selected for a biological test." "Clove essential oil can be considered as a potential antimicrobial agent for external use". "Dormans and Deans (6) evaluated the antibacterial activity of six essential oils against 25 different genera of bacteria; all bacteria had a degree of sensitivity to essential oils tested. Oils with higher activity were thyme, oregano and cloves." The parenthesised 6 is one of the references listed at the end of "Microbicide activity of clove essential oil (Eugenia caryophyllata)"; ordinarily I would leave out other paper's references, but this entire quote references that other study. "The high levels of eugenol contained in clove essential oil are responsible for its strong biological and antimicrobial activities. It is well know that both eugenol and clove essential oil phenolic compounds can denature proteins and react with cell membrane phospholipids changing their permeability and inhibiting a great number of Gram-negative and Gram-positive bacteria as well as different types of yeast". Figure 1 does a remarkable job at displaying the antibacterial ability of Clove EO. 37 celsius is equal to 98.6 fahrenheit (the average of healthy body temperature): "The inactivation kinetics depends on the temperature. Those results show that bacteria inactivation was more effective at a higher temperature (37°C), thus the temperature coefficient calculation shows that at 37°C the activity is 18 to 19 times higher than a 21°C, depending on the microorganism. This activity increase must be considered in the application of clove essential oil as antiseptic."

Citation: Nuñez L, Aquino MD. Microbicide activity of clove essential oil (Eugenia caryophyllata). Braz J Microbiol. 2012 Oct;43(4):1255-60. doi: 10.1590/S1517-83822012000400003. Epub 2012 Jun 1. PMID: 24031950; PMCID: PMC3769004.

Title: Antibacterial activity of plant extracts and phytochemicals on antibiotic-resistant bacteria

URL:
https://www.scielo.br/j/bjm/a/tLgk49SrVLgtNJqG9z7SSsR/abstract/?lang=en

Authors: Gislene G. F. Nascimento; Juliana Locatelli; Paulo C. Freitas; Giuliana L. Silva

MY Summary: This is a very basic overview of a primary study investigating the antibacterial action of 10 essential oils: Yarrow, Clove, Lemon-balm, Basil, Guava, Pomegranate, Rosemary, Sage, Jambolan, and Thyme. Clove oil was the best general antimicrobial with it successfully inhibiting 64.2% of the tested microorganisms (9 out of 14 with minimum inhibition zone of 7mm), and Jambolan was in 2nd place with 57.1% (8 out of 14 with minimum inhibition zone of 7mm). Clove was classified as effective against Staphylococcus aureus, Salmonella choleraesuis, Pseudomonas aeruginosa, Candida albicans, Klebsiella pneumoniae (drug resistant) at 0.01% concentration, Klebsiella pneumoniae (super drug resistant) at 0.01% concentration, Shigella (drug resistant) at .025% concentration, Proteus (drug resistant) at 0.002% concentration, and Pseudomonas aeruginosa (super drug resistant) at .005% concentration; of note, the last 5 of the listed bacteria were obtained from hospitals local to Brazil. None of the 10 essential oils were classified as successful against Escherichia coli (drug resistant) with as much concentration as 0.05%.

Citation: Nascimento, G. G. F., Locatelli, J., Freitas, P. C., & Silva, G. L.. (2000). Antibacterial activity of plant extracts and phytochemicals on antibiotic-resistant bacteria. Brazilian Journal of Microbiology, 31(Braz. J. Microbiol., 2000 31(4)). https://doi.org/10.1590/S1517-83822000000400003

Title: Mechanism of Action of Topical Garlic on Wound Healing

URL: https://pubmed.ncbi.nlm.nih.gov/29077629/

Authors: Minhal Alhashim; Jamie Lombardo

MY Summary: This is a primary study. The primary active component of Garlic - Allicin - increases the proliferation of fibroblasts in wounds to speed up healing. Also, allicin is a strong antimicrobial.

Citation: Alhashim M, Lombardo J. Mechanism of Action of Topical Garlic on Wound Healing. Dermatol Surg. 2018 May;44(5):630-634. doi: 10.1097/DSS.0000000000001382. PMID: 29077629.

Title: Antibacterial Properties of Organosulfur Compounds of Garlic (Allium sativum)

URL: https://www.ncbi.nlm.nih.gov/pmc/articles/PMC8362743/

Authors: Sushma Bagde Bhatwalkar; Rajesh Mondal; Suresh Babu Naidu Krishna; Jamila Khatoon Adam; Patrick Govender; Rajaneesh Anupam

MY Summary: This paper goes over the antimicrobial action of the several forms of garlic use, from simply cutting it, to drying it, to soaking it in water, ethanol, or acetone, to specific components, to its earlier active components, to its later-stage primary active components, and even to co-admission of antimicrobial drugs. If you wish to read this paper specifically about use of garlic in my book, take special note of the sections "Antibacterial Activity of Garlic Aqueous Extract" and "Antibacterial Activity of Ajoene" as these two sections most closely encapsulate the actions of garlic in the salves.

Citation: Bhatwalkar SB, Mondal R, Krishna SBN, Adam JK, Govender P, Anupam R. Antibacterial Properties of Organosulfur Compounds of Garlic (Allium sativum). Front Microbiol. 2021 Jul 27;12:613077. doi: 10.3389/fmicb.2021.613077. PMID: 34394014; PMCID: PMC8362743.

Title: Antimicrobial properties of allicin from garlic

URL: https://pubmed.ncbi.nlm.nih.gov/10594976/

Authors: S Ankri; D Mirelman

MY Summary: This was only a 1 paragraph abstract, which states that allicin itself is against a wide variety of bacteria, including multidrug resistant ones, fungi, parasites, and viruses.

Citation: Ankri S, Mirelman D. Antimicrobial properties of allicin from garlic. 1Microbes Infect. 1999 Feb;1(2):125-9. doi: 10.1016/s1286-4579(99)80003-3. PMID: 10594976.

Title: Allicin Reduces the Production of α-Toxin by Staphylococcus aureus

URL: https://www.ncbi.nlm.nih.gov/pmc/articles/PMC6264299/

Authors: Bing-Feng Leng,1,† Jia-Zhang Qiu,1,† Xiao-Han Dai,1,† Jing Dong,1 Jian-Feng Wang; Ming-Jing Luo; Hong-En Li; Xiao-Di Niu; Yu Zhang; Yong-Xing Ai; Xu-Ming Deng

MY Summary: The abstract: "Staphylococcus aureus causes a broad range of life-threatening diseases in humans. The pathogenicity of this micro-organism is largely dependent upon its virulence factors [virus or bacteria created compounds that assist the virus or bacteria to further infect the host]. One of the most extensively studied virulence factors is the extracellular protein α-toxin. In this study, we show that allicin, an organosulfur compound, was active against S. aureus with MICs [Minimum Inhibitory Concentrations] [ranging] from 32 to 64 μg/mL [0.0032% to 0.0064% concentration]. Haemolysis, Western blot and real-time RT-PCR assays [types of super-specialized examination tests] were used to evaluate the effects of allicin on S. aureus α-toxin production and on the levels of gene expression [the level of activity of a gene], respectively. The results of our study indicated that sub-inhibitory concentrations [below 0.0032% concentration] of allicin decreased the production of α-toxin in both methicillin-sensitive S. aureus (MSSA) and methicillin-resistant S. aureus (MRSA) in a dose-dependent manner. Furthermore, the transcriptional levels of agr (accessory gene regulator) in S. aureus were inhibited by allicin. Therefore, allicin may be useful in the treatment of α-toxin-producing S. aureus infections." After the abstract, it talks specifically about Staphylococcus Aureus, and then gives details of the test results. Next it explains the potential impact of allicin on the drug-resistant S. Aureus, which has been rapidly growing and is revealing itself as a direct danger that is also becoming more difficult to treat by current pharmaceutical methods. Then it gives the details of the procedures for the experiments and follows with a brief conclusion.

Citation: Leng BF, Qiu JZ, Dai XH, Dong J, Wang JF, Luo MJ, Li HE, Niu XD, Zhang Y, Ai YX, Deng XM. Allicin reduces the production of α-toxin by Staphylococcus aureus. Molecules. 2011

Sep 15;16(9):7958-68. doi: 10.3390/molecules16097958. PMID: 21921868; PMCID: PMC6264299.

Title: Overview of wound healing in a moist environment

URL: https://pubmed.ncbi.nlm.nih.gov/8109679/

Authors: F K Field; M D Kerstein

MY Summary: One key sentence in the one paragraph abstract: "The beneficial effects of a moist versus a dry wound environment include: prevention of tissue dehydration and cell death, accelerated angiogenesis, increased breakdown of dead tissue and fibrin, i.e., pericapillary fibrin cuffs, and potentiating the interaction of growth factors with their target cells."

Citation: Field FK, Kerstein MD. Overview of wound healing in a moist environment. Am J Surg. 1994 Jan;167(1A):2S-6S. doi: 10.1016/0002-9610(94)90002-7. PMID: 8109679.

Title: A Rapid Review of Burns First Aid Guidelines: Is There Consistency Across International Guidelines?

URL: https://www.ncbi.nlm.nih.gov/pmc/articles/PMC8291991/

Authors: Michael McLure; Finlay Macneil; Fiona M Wood; Leila Cuttle; Kathryn Eastwood; Janet Bray; Lincoln M Tracy

MY Summary: "The World Health Organization (WHO) defines burns as 'an injury to the skin or other organic tissue primarily caused by heat or due to radiation, radioactivity, electricity, friction or chemicals' " (I changed the quote's quote into apostrophes). "In the case of burns, studies have demonstrated that the early application of appropriate first aid improves patient outcomes following injury.

Improved patient outcomes associated with cool water first aid treatment include a reduction in burn depth, faster re-epithelialization, lower rates of grafting or less body surface area being grafted, shorter hospital length of stay, and significantly decreased rates of intensive care unit admission."

Citation: McLure M, Macneil F, Wood FM, Cuttle L, Eastwood K, Bray J, Tracy LM. A Rapid Review of Burns First Aid Guidelines: Is There Consistency Across International Guidelines? Cureus. 2021 Jun 20;13(6):e15779. doi: 10.7759/cureus.15779. PMID: 34295589; PMCID: PMC8291991.

Title: Common bacterial skin infections

URL: https://pubmed.ncbi.nlm.nih.gov/12126026/

Authors: Daniel L Stulberg; Marc A Penrod; Richard A Blatny

MY Summary: The most common bacterial skin infections are from Streptococcus and Staphylococcus bacteria species.

Citation: Stulberg DL, Penrod MA, Blatny RA. Common bacterial skin infections. Am Fam Physician. 2002 Jul 1;66(1):119-24. PMID: 12126026.

Title: Microbial Species Isolated from Infected Wounds and Antimicrobial Resistance Analysis: Data Emerging from a Three-Years Retrospective Study

URL: https://www.ncbi.nlm.nih.gov/pmc/articles/PMC8532735/ .

Authors: Valentina Puca; Roberta Zita Marulli; Rossella Grande; Irene Vitale; Antonietta Niro; Gina Molinaro; Silvia Prezioso; Raffaella Muraro; Pamela Di Giovanni

MY Summary: This was a retrospective study of hospital-treated infections for years 2017, 2018, and 2019 from a single hospital in Italy. About 40% of infections occurred inside of the hospital while about 60% occurred outside of the hospital. Almost 25% of the treated infections were infected by 2 or more microbes, making it a much more difficult and dangerous infection; there were 239 wounds with 59 of them being infected by multiple microbes (the 59 multi-infections averaged 2.2 microbes). The bacteria or fungi present in at least 1% of infections were *[B: G-Pos is Bacteria Gram Positive; B: G-Neg is Bacteria Gram Negative; F is Fungus]*: (B: G-Pos) Staphylococcus aureus 29.13%, (B: G-Neg) Pseudomonas aeruginosa 23.30%, (B: G-Neg) Escherichia coli 11.97%, (B: G-Neg) Proteus mirabilis 6.47%, (B: G-Neg) Acinetobacter baumannii/haemolyticus 5.50%, (B: G-Neg) Serratia marcescens 2.27%, (F) Candida albicans 2.27%, (B: G-Neg) Enterobacter cloacae 1.94%, (B: G-Neg) Klebsiella pneumoniae 1.62%, (B: G-Neg) Morganella morganii 1.62%, and (B: G-Pos) Staphylococcus haemolyticus 1.62%. The remainder were: (B: G-Neg) Alcaligenes 0.97%, (B: G-Pos) Enterococcus faecalis 0.97%, (B: G-Pos) Staphylococcus epidermidis 0.97%, (F) Candida glabrata 0.97%, (F) Candida parapsilosis 0.97%, (B: G-Neg) Citrobacter freundii 0.65%, (B: G-Neg) Providencia 0.65%, (B: G-Pos) Staphylococcus auricularis 0.65%, (B: G-Pos) Staphylococcus lugdunensis 0.65%, (B: G-Pos) Staphylococcus simulans 0.65%, (B: G-Neg) Klebsiella ornithinolytica 0.32%, (B: G-Neg) Proteus vulgaris 0.32%, (B: G-Neg) Pseudomonas fluorescens/putida 0.32%, (B: G-Pos) Enterococcus avium 0.32%, (B: G-Pos) Staphylococcus schleiferi subsp. coagulans 0.32%, (B: G-Pos) Staphylococcus sciuri 0.32%, (B: G-Pos) Streptococcus agalactiae 0.32%, (B: G-Pos) Streptococcus pyogenes 0.32%, (B: G-Pos) Streptococcus salivarius 0.32%, (F) Candida guilliermondii 0.32%, (F) Candida stellatoidea 0.32%, (F) Candida tropicalis 0.32%, and (F) Candida 0.32%. Almost 9 in 10 of these infections were resistant to at least 1 antibiotic, and as many as 29.2% were resistant to at least 6 different antibiotics. " The WHO report of 2014 indicates that multi-drug resistant pathogens are responsible for about 25,000 death and 23,000 death every year in Europe and the United States, respectively. Moreover, about the 50% of infections associated with E. coli, K. pneumoniae, S. aureus and P. aeruginosa showed resistance against the most effective antimicrobials such as third-generation cephalosporin". To help emphasize the resources that directly talk about the microbes in over 1% of the studied infections, they have all been highlighted.

Citation: Puca V, Marulli RZ, Grande R, Vitale I, Niro A, Molinaro G, Prezioso S, Muraro R, Di Giovanni P. Microbial Species Isolated from Infected Wounds and Antimicrobial Resistance Analysis: Data Emerging from a Three-Years Retrospective Study. Antibiotics (Basel). 2021 Sep 24;10(10):1162. doi: 10.3390/antibiotics10101162. PMID: 34680743; PMCID: PMC8532735.

Title: Wound healing: cellular mechanisms and pathological outcomes

URL: https://www.ncbi.nlm.nih.gov/pmc/articles/PMC7536089/

Authors: Holly N. Wilkinson; Matthew J. Hardman

MY Summary: This educational paper first goes into great detail about the wound repair process, directly explaining even the minute actions of specific cell types, the phases they are involved in, etc. Next it details what changes old age and also diabetes cause that impair the wound healing process. After that, it goes into detail about various advances beginning to take place to improve our ability to study and understand the skin and especially the wound healing process itself.

Then it addresses risk of infection and the importance of developing targeted antibacterial techniques that preserve the commensal and symbiotic bacteria while targeting the harmful microbes; it also somewhat discusses developing drug resistance of these harmful microbes. Two of the sentences in the ending conclusion does well in explaining the purpose of this educational paper: "The high cellular diversity, complexity and plasticity of wound healing provide a considerable challenge to comprehensively elucidate. While this remains a perplexing goal, it is essential that we continue to strive to more fully understand the mechanisms that underpin both normal and pathological healing."

Citation: Wilkinson HN, Hardman MJ. Wound healing: cellular mechanisms and pathological outcomes. Open Biol. 2020 Sep;10(9):200223. doi: 10.1098/rsob.200223. Epub 2020 Sep 30. PMID: 32993416; PMCID: PMC7536089.

Printed in the USA
CPSIA information can be obtained
at www.ICGtesting.com
JSHW010816051223
52884JS00013B/229